CELLULAR SIGNALS CONTROLLING UTERINE FUNCTION

CELLULAR SIGNALS CONTROLLING UTERINE FUNCTION

Edited by

Lynn A. Lavia

Wichita State University
Wichita, Kansas

PLENUM PRESS • NEW YORK AND LONDON

Library of Congress Cataloging-in-Publication Data

Symposium on Cellular Signals Controlling Uterine Function (1989 :
  Wichita, Kan.)
    Cellular signals controlling uterine function / edited by Lynn
  A. Lavia.
        p.   cm.
    "Proceedings of a Symposium on Cellular Signals Controlling
  Uterine Function, held September 21-22, 1989, in Wichita, Kansas"-
  -T.p. verso.
    Includes bibliographical references and index.
    ISBN 0-306-43822-4
    1. Uterus--Physiology--Congresses. 2. Cellular signal
  transduction--Congresses. 3. Growth factors--Physiological effect-
  -Congresses. 4. Cytokines--Physiological effect--Congresses.
  I. Lavia, Lynn A. II. Title.
    [DNLM: 1. Cell Communication--physiology--congresses. 2. Signal
  Transduction--physiology--congresses. 3. Uterus--cytology-
  -congresses.   WP 400 S9885c]
  QP262.S94   1989
  612.6'2--dc20
  DNLM/DLC
  for Library of Congress   91-2474
                                                               CIP

Proceedings of a Symposium on Cellular Signals Controlling Uterine
Function, held September 21–22, 1989, in Wichita, Kansas

ISBN 0-306-43822-4

© 1991 Plenum Press, New York
A Division of Plenum Publishing Corporation
233 Spring Street, New York, N.Y. 10013

Printed in the United States of America

Contents

1

Prologue

Endocrine hormone signals are known to act on the uterine target organ by inducing specific paracrine interactions between populations of cells within this marvelous incubator of the world. This Symposium was organized to bring together scientists with acumen in various areas of cell biology who have chosen to study the uterus as their model. The idea was to exchange information on cellular signaling which affect three major areas of uterine biology. The major themes addressed by the Symposium included: 1) signals responsible for ontogenetic and phylogenetic uterine morphogenesis and growth; 2) signals required for successful implantation and embryonic growth, as well as; 3) signals required for the genetic programming of normal and abnormal uterine growth. The Symposium was held on September 21-22, 1989, in Wichita Kansas. The Symposium attracted over 150 participants, these included scientists and students from the United States as well as some from abroad.

The organizers wish to thank for the wide support for this conference, provided both by the University of Kansas School of Medicine, and The Wichita State University Department of Biological Sciences. A special thanks to Dr. William Reals, Ms. Ginger Ewonus, and Ms. Judy Sparks, from the University of Kansas School of Medicine-Wichita, who assisted in preparations for the conference. Thanks also goes to my good friend, Dr. Brett A. Larson of Wichita State, who was my co-chair and helped immensely. A special thanks also goes to Ms. Diedre Martin and Ms. Pamela Flaming, who did outstanding jobs in assisting with the preparation of this book. The conference was made possible by a generous grant from The Wesley Foundation, with additional support from Sheerin Scientific Company, Inc., Jacobs Instrument Company, Inc. and Ortho Pharmaceutical Corporation.

The Symposium was held in honor of Dr. Howard A. Bern, Professor of Integrative Biology and Research Endocrinologist in the Cancer Research Laboratory at the University of California, Berkeley. Dr. Bern has not only done an extensive amount of research in comparative and uterine endocrinology, as well as in cancer, but has also trained an outstanding number of excellent researchers in these areas. Introductory remarks by Dr. Gil Greenwald of the University of Kansas School of Medicine-Kansas City, below, highlight Howard's remarkable achievements.

Introduction of Professor Bern

I was overjoyed when Dr. Lavia invited me to present some introductory remarks about Dr. Howard Bern because, like so many people in this room, I consider him my scientific blood brother. Howard has had a most fulfilling and productive career, both as a scientist and as a man. He received his Ph.D. from U.C.L.A. in 1948, and then joined the staff at the Department of Zoology at Berkeley as an instructor. Yes, Virginia, believe it or not, in those days, people actually were hired as instructors. He rose rapidly through the ranks, was promoted to Assistant Professor in 1950 and Professor in 1960. Currently he is Professor of Integrated Biology, Research Endocrinologist at the Cancer Research Bureau and Chief of the Endocrinology Group at Berkeley. His accomplishments are too numerous to elaborate, but three that I think he is most proud of are his election to the National Academy of Sciences in 1975; his membership of the American Academy of Arts and Sciences, and past-president of the American Society of Zoology in 1967.

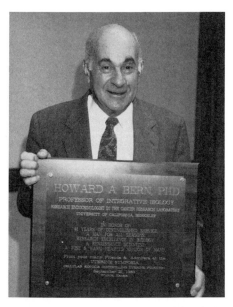

Figure 1. Professor Howard Bern after receiving his honorary plaque at the Symposium.

The next figures are truly mind boggling. In his unusually productive career he has had over 90 postdoctoral and visiting professors working in his laboratory; it is a veritable U.N. with students and colleagues throughout the world. In addition, he has trained as the major professor 44 Ph.D. students with three gestating at this very moment.

As a result of this tremendous interaction with so many people, Howard has published over 370 papers. The publications are significant not only in terms of their number but also in the quality of work. I have a fair sprinkling of his publications and I went back and pulled out some of the early ones that came out during the 50's and 60's as they represent the thematic threads that have recurred throughout his research career.

For example, one paper is entitled *The taxonomic specificity of prolactin*, that he did with Carl Nicoll. This is one of his major interests: comparative aspects of prolactin. Another paper is *The cytochemical studies of cytokeratin formation and epithelial metaplasia in the rodent vagina;* an example of a long term interest in the hormonal factors regulating the vaginal epithelium. Another paper is entitled *Cytochemical studies of hyperplastic alveolar nodules in the mammary gland of the mouse,* published along with Max Alfert. Tumor biology and mammary tumors, in particular, is another *leit motiv.* Finally, one called *Electrophysiologic indications of the osmoregulatory role of the teleost urophysis;* the neurosecretory system at both the cranial and caudal ends of animals is a persistent topic. In perusing these papers I've made a list of species that his laboratory has utilized. This is just a small fraction, and I'm sure it could be enlarged considerably. His research group has worked with rabbits, mice, rats, guinea pigs, toads, frogs, sea lions, octopus, passerine birds, leeches, teleost fishes, and last but not least, the male wormbeetle *Tenebrio.* Howard is truly a comparative endocrinologist whose research covers the gamut of invertebrate and vertebrate species.

These are the cold facts that can be gleaned from his C.V. But having known him for over 40 years, bonding long ago when he was a young professor at Berkeley and I was a neophyte, bushy-tailed graduate student, I think I'd like to flesh out this account with some recollections of Howard in the early years. First of all, a trait that he has always exhibited is his tremendous enthusiasm and spontaneity. Howard is a superb lecturer. In his course in Endocrinology, quite frequently, right before lecturing he could be found ensconced in one of his favorite habitats: the Life Sciences library. Howard is an omnivorous reader and he was always devouring the latest journals. Consequently, quite often he would burst into class and launch into a tangent, completely veering from the topic of the day, because he had just read something that aroused his enthusiasm because of the experimental design, the topic or the elegance of the work.

Another trait is his boundless energy. I've never seen Howard walk. He moves slightly less than the speed of light. You have to get out of his way if you were walking through the corridors; he always seems to be going someplace, always with some mission in life which has to be fulfilled in the next five minutes.

Friendliness: If you ever go to a national meeting where Howard is present, sooner or later he acts like a magnet. Everyone gravitates to his vicinity. It doesn't make any difference whether you're a first year graduate student or a senior colleague which he has known for many years. This is one of his major attributes: His openness and ability to interact with people under any circumstance.

One of Howard's characteristics, appropriate to this symposium, is his trepidation before lectures whether to a class or the presentation which he will shortly deliver. It's not a matter of nervousness; it's a necessary build up of tension. Howard's like a high-spirited race horse waiting to get out of the starter's gate. He needs that period of nervousness beforehand in order to perform up to snuff. He once confided to Dr. Richard Goldschmidt that he usually had to spend a few minutes in the bathroom before lecturing. Goldschmidt was a very dignified, distinguished Professor of Genetics at Berkeley, rather frosty and intimidating to most graduate students. Goldschmidt replied that although he was 80 he still experienced the same symptoms before lecturing!!

I could go on and on about Professor Bern, but only a few moments are left. If permitted I could regale you with the story about his discovery of sex at an early age in Montreal; this will have to wait for tonight's reception. In summary, Howard is indeed a superb scholar, gentleman and family man. These are hackneyed expressions, but hackneyed expressions have a way of being true. The day before I coming here Wichita, I was cleaning up my bulletin board and found a tattered, yellowing clipping posted years ago. It was Aristotle's concept of the ideal or the "great-souled" man, and as I looked at it, it was apparent that Aristotle knew Howard Bern!! Aristotle concludes:

> *...to be truly great-minded a man must be good and whatever is great in each virtue would seem to belong to the great-minded. In wealth, in power, in good or bad fortune of every kind he will bear himself with moderation. He is the sort of man to do kindness. Further, it is characteristic of the great-minded man not to ask favors or very reluctantly, but to do service very readily. He is open in his likes and dislikes, cares more for reality than appearance and speaks the truth. He is not servile in the presence of the great or wealthy nor condescending toward people of middle station.*

That last statement epitomizes Howard.   His accomplishments in science are truly impressive. I could go on and on in terms of the invited lectures he has given, the committees he has served on. But I think the fact that he lacks hubris, that he has risen to his stature without stepping over people, without rancor, with a great openness of spirit, truly exemplifies this extraordinary man. In his honor his students have prepared a plaque. The inscription reads:

Howard A. Bern, Ph.D.
Professor of Integrative Biology
Research Endocrinologist in the Cancer Research Laboratory
University of California, Berkeley
In Honor of 41 Years of Distinguished Service
A man for All Seasons
Research Excellence in Biology
A Renaissance Scientist
A Wise and Warm-Hearted Mentor of Many
From your many Friends and Admirers at the Uterine Symposium
September 21, 1989

2

Is Estrogen a Cellular Signal for Female Genital Tract Epithelium?

Howard A. Bern (with the collaboration of F.-D. A. Uchima, T. Iguchi, P.-S. Tsai and M. Edery)
Department of Integrative Biology and Cancer Research Laboratory
University of California
Berkeley, California 94720

Summary

In vivo, the vagina and uterus, and their respective epithelial linings, are considered to be estrogen target structures. As a result of classical endocrinological studies, their dependence on estrogen for growth and differentiation is considered axiomatic. *In vitro*, primary cultures of epithelial cells from the vagina and uterus, grown in collagen gel matrix in a serum-free medium, proliferate independently of the presence of added estrogen. Addition of estrogen to these primary cultures does not stimulate epithelial cell proliferation, even in suboptimal conditions, but rather retards their growth. The estrogen receptor system of these cultured cells appears to be functionally intact, and the cells respond to estrogen addition by specific product synthesis (progestin receptors). Thus, estrogen has a direct modulative effect on cultured vaginal and uterine epithelia, but estrogen is not a directly-acting mitogen for these cells. It appears that stromal and possibly organismal factors are essential synergists and/or mediators for estrogen's well-known mitogenic effect on female genital epithelia *in vivo*. Several alternative pathways for estrogen action on female genital epithelia are suggested.

Introduction

The vagina and uterus are archetypical target organs for the action of estrogen. It has been axiomatic that the growth and function of the epithelium lining these organs are directly stimulated by estrogen. This axiom is based on years of experimentation *in vivo*. The present report is concerned with the degree to which estrogen is a direct signal to the vaginal and endometrial epithelia.

Methodological Comments

Over the past ten years, our laboratory has developed the primary culture of vaginal and uterine (luminal) epithelial cells in a defined serum-free medium, using collagen gel matrix (6-8). Both the initial medium and the collagen gel methodology are essentially those employed in the sister laboratory of our colleague S. Nandi and his associates (21). Isolated cells will proliferate when placed upon or when embedded in collagen gel; in most experiments referred to herein, we have observed three-dimensional growth inside the collagen gel matrix.

Vagina and uterus are subjected to enzymatic dissociation with collagenase and with trypsin, respectively. DNase treatment is used to help remove cell debris. A Percoll gradient step was later introduced to aid in cell separation and to protect steroid receptors. All mice were females of the BALB/cCrgl strain, initially about 35 days old when ovariectomized and about 40 days old when killed (to minimize the effect of endogenous estrogen). However, it has proven more convenient and economical to use intact 21-day-old (prepuberal) mice as a tissue source (K. T. Mills, C. Wong and H. A. Bern, unpublished). The serum-free complete (SFc) medium routinely employed is a 1:1 mixture of Dulbecco's modification of Eagle's medium and Ham's F12 medium, supplemented with insulin (10 μg/ml), epidermal growth factor (EGF: 10 ng/ml), bovine serum albumin fraction V (BSA: 5 mg/ml), transferrin (10 μg/ml), cholera toxin (10 ng/ml) and antibiotics, presently buffered with HEPES. A second medium (SF20) lacking cholera toxin, which appears to be dispensable, has been used with the prepuberal cell cultures.

Findings

Several criteria were employed to confirm the epithelial nature of the cultured cells. For the vaginal cultures, these included electron-microscope demonstration of tonofibrils and desmosomes, the ability to form a pluristratified epithelium when cultured on collagen gel and to generate superficial keratin when the gels were detached (floating gels), immuno-cytochemical demonstration of keratin (6,8), and ability to form a typical hormone-responsive vaginal epithelium when cultures were recombined with an appropriate stroma and transplanted under the renal capsule of an athymic nude mouse (2). When vaginae from prepuberal mice are used, stratification and keratinization occur in colonies in the gel (18). For the endometrial cultures, criteria were ultrastructure and behavior on transplantation (2,7).

Vaginal epithelial cells increase in number in SFc medium multifold during 10 days in culture without added estrogen (17β-estradiol or diethylstilbestrol). Thus, estrogen is not a requirement for vaginal epithelial cell proliferation *in vitro* in our system (6,8). The possibility existed that the medium used (SFc or SF20) was supportive of maximal proliferation; hence, no additional stimulation by estrogen could be expected. However, when suboptimal (insulin, EGF, BSA) or minimal (insulin, BSA) media were used, growth of vaginal epithelial cells still occurred, albeit much less, but estrogen again was unable to stimulate proliferation (6,8). It is important to emphasize that all our cultures referred to herein were conducted in the absence of serum. Interesting and sometimes different findings have been reported when serum supplements are used. However, it is difficult to estimate the contribution of known and unknown factors in the serum to the results obtained.

Concern could be raised as to whether the cultured epithelial cells, growing independently of estrogen, were a selected cell population and no longer normal vaginal cells. When such cell cultures were transplanted into nude mice (see above), they disappeared and did not produce any abnormal growths. However, when such cultures were combined with normal vaginal stroma and transplanted, the cells proliferated as vaginal epithelium, responding to the host's cyclical ovarian hormone production, to ovariectomy, and to estrogen replacement therapy in a typical fashion (2). Transplanted uterine epithelial cultures also responded appropriately to the host's hormonal milieu (2).

Questions about the integrity of the estrogen receptor system raised further concern. However, cultured cells showed both estrogen and progestin receptors, the former admittedly in relatively small numbers in vaginal cells. Both vaginal and endometrial luminal cells responded to the addition of appropriate quantities of 17β-estradiol to the culture medium by a decrease in cytosolic estrogen binding, an increase in nuclear estrogen binding, and a notable increase in progestin binding (19,20; see also 17). These experiments established two important points: First, estrogen receptors were present and functionally responsive, and second, both vaginal and endometrial cells were responsive to estrogen in terms of specific product synthesis (progestin receptors), even though they remained mitotically non-responsive.

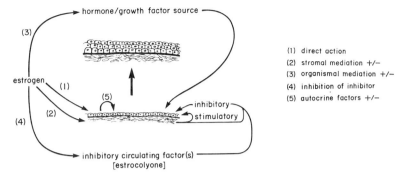

Figure 1. Estrogen and other chemical mediators as possible signals in the female genital tract. See text for discussion.

In other words, although estrogen was not a direct mitogen for the female genital tract epithelium, it was still acting as a steroid hormone in regard to progestin receptor induction.

When prepuberal vaginal cells are cultured in the absence of estrogen, quasi-normal differentiation also occurs: enlargement and sloughing of superficial mucous-appearing cells and keratinization of cells underlying the mucous cell layer (18). These changes are also not affected by estrogen addition (18). Thus, both proliferation and differentiation of isolated vaginal epithelium appear to be estrogen-independent in our system.

Although estrogen does not stimulate mitosis directly in our system, it does inhibit mitosis in a dose-related fashion (6-8, 18-20). This effect appears to be specific to estrane derivatives (18) or to synthetic estrogens such as diethylstilbestrol (6,8), and its action on cell cultures can best be described as exerting a retardation effect on cell growth. The antiestrogen keoxifene interferes with the ability of 17β-estradiol to exert this retardation, again in a dose-related fashion (18,19).

Implications

Estrogen does not appear to be a direct signal for mitogenesis of vaginal and endometrial epithelia in our system of primary culture in serum-free media. Similarly-cultured mammary epithelium is also not responsive to added estrogen in terms of proliferation (9). Other studies of cultured endometrial epithelial cells also indicate a lack of mitotic response to estrogen unless stroma is also present (10).

Figure 1 attempts to present alternative pathways by which estrogen may act on female genital tract epithelia, judging from analytic studies on rodent models. First, estrogen may affect the epithelium directly. This appears to be true in regard to specific product synthesis (e.g., progestin receptor) and to retardation of proliferation. The retardation could be mediated by local production of an inhibitory growth factor such as transforming growth factor-β (see 11,17 and pathway 5, Figure 1). Second, estrogen may act upon the stroma to cause the production of a stimulatory mitogenic factor (2-4). The non-responsiveness of cultured epithelial cells to added estrogen and the non-proliferation (non-retrieval) of cultured cells transplanted into a host without stromal contact support this explanation. However, the ability of epithelial cells to proliferate in culture independently of stroma and of estrogen raises the possibility of the production of a mitosis-inhibitory factor by the stroma. Estrogen would then act on the stroma to inhibit the production of this inhibitor (cf. 12). Third, it is possible that systemic hormones and/or growth factors are produced *in vivo* under the influence of estrogen, which modulate the proliferative activity of the genital epithelial cells. Pituitary hormones such as prolactin or distantly-produced growth factors (estromedins) are candidates for agents in such a pathway. This kind of reasoning has been extensively developed by Sirbasku and his colleagues (13,14). Addition of prolactin, alone or with estrogen, to our vaginal cultures was not mitogenic, however (8). Fourth, the existence of a circulating inhibitor of mitosis in estrogen-dependent organs has been proposed by Sonnenschein and Soto and their associates (15,16). The binding of estrogen to this factor(s) would functionally inactivate it and thus relieve the inhibition over proliferation. Fifth, local factors may operate by autocrine mechanisms (see 1,5,11,14,17). Thus, the dissociation of the epithelium from its normal organotypic relations may result in the production of locally active growth factors (such as epidermal growth factor), and these "injured" cells would thus support their own proliferation. Tsai (18) has recently found increased epithelial mitotic activity at the cut ends of organ-cultured vaginae, compared with more central areas, raising the possibility of a local "wound repair" mechanism.

In summary, experiments with primary cultures of normal vaginal and uterine epithelial cells have led to a series of unexpected and even paradoxical observations, leading to the unavoidable conclusion that the "cellular signals controlling" female genital tract growth and function are complex both in reality and in possibility.

Acknowledgments

The research from our laboratory has been aided by National Institutes of Health Grants CA-05388 and CA-09041. In recent years, we wish to acknowledge particularly the help of Karen Tanada Mills and Calvin Wong in the development of the culture system using prepuberal mice, Susan Hamamoto for electron microscopy and immunocytochemistry, Naomi Lidicker for histology, John Underhill for photography, Phyllis Spowart for figure preparation, and Srisawai Pattamakom and Ken Takemura for important laboratory assistance.

References

1. Buckley, A., Davidson, J.M., Kamerath, C.D., Wolt, T.B., and Woodward, S.C., Sustained release of epidermal growth factor accelerates wound repair, Proc. Natl. Acad. Sci. USA, 82:7340 (1985).
2. Cooke, P.S., Uchima, F.-D.A., Fujii, D.K., Bern, H.A., and Cunha, G.R., Restoration of normal morphology and estrogen responsiveness in cultured vaginal and uterine epithelia transplanted with stroma, Proc. Natl. Acad. Sci. USA, 83:2109 (1986).
3. Cunha, G.R., Stromal induction and specification of morphogenesis and cytodifferentiation of the epithelia of the Mullerian ducts and urogenital sinus during development of the uterus and vagina in mice, J. Exp. Zool., 196:361 (1976).
4. Cunha, G.R. and Fujii, H., Stromal-parenchymal interactions in normal and abnormal development of the genital tract, In: *Developmental Effects of Diethylstilbestrol (DES) in Pregnancy*, A.L. Herbst and H.A. Bern, (eds.), Thieme-Stratton, New York (1981).
5. Gilchrest, B.A., Karassik, R.L., Wilkins, L.M., Vrabel, M.A., and Maciag, T., Autocrine and paracrine growth stimulation of cells derived from human skin, J. Cell. Physiol., 117:235-240.
6. Iguchi, T., Uchima, F.-D.A., Ostrander, P.L., and Bern, H.A., Growth of normal mouse vaginal epithelial cells in and on collagen gels, Proc. Natl. Acad. Sci. USA, 80:3743 (1983).
7. Iguchi, T., Uchima, F.-D.A., Ostrander, P.L., Hamamoto, S.T., and Bern, H.A., Proliferation of normal mouse uterine luminal epithelial cells in serum-free collagen gel culture, Proc. Japan Acad., 61B:292 (1985).
8. Iguchi, T., Uchima, F.-D.A., and Bern, H.A., Growth of mouse vaginal epithelial cells in culture: effect of sera and supplemented serum-free media. *In Vitro* Cell. Devel. Biol., 23:535 (1987).
9. Imagawa, W., Tomooka, Y., and Nandi, S., Serum-free growth of normal and tumor mouse mammary epithelial cells in primary culture, Proc. Natl. Acad. Sci. USA, 79:4074 (1982).

10. Inaba, T., Wiest, W.G., Strickler, R.C., and Mori, J., Augmentation of the response of mouse uterine epithelial cells to estradiol by uterine stroma, Endocrinology, 123:1253 (1988).

11. Knabbe, C., Lippman, M.E., Wakefield, L.M., Flanders, K.C., Kasid, A., Derynck, R., and Dickson R.B., Evidence that transforming growth factor-β is a hormonally regulated negative growth factor in human breast cancer cells, Cell, 48:417 (1987).

12. Shafie, S.M., Estrogen and the growth of breast cancer: new evidence suggests indirect action, Science, 209:701 (1980).

13. Sirbasku, D.A., Estrogen induction of growth factors specific for hormone-responsive mammary, pituitary, and kidney tumor cells, Proc. Natl. Acad. Sci. USA, 75:3786 (1978).

14. Sirbasku, D.A., Ikeda, T., and Danielpour, D., Characterization of endocrine and autocrine mammary tumor cell growth factors, In: *Growth and Differentiation of Cells in Defined Environment*, H. Murakami., (eds.), Springer-Verlag, Berlin (1985).

15. Soto, A.M. and Sonnenschein, C., The role of estrogens on the proliferation of human breast tumor cells (MCF-7), J. Steroid Biochem., 23:87 (1985).

16. Soto, A.M. and Sonnenschein, C., Cell proliferation of estrogen-sensitive cells: The case for negative control, Endocrine Rev., 8:44-52 (1987).

17. Sumida, C., Lecerf, F., and Pasqualini, J.R., Control of progesterone receptors in fetal uterine cells in culture: effects of estradiol, progestins, antiestrogens, and growth factors, Endocrinology, 122:3 (1988).

18. Tsai, P.-S., Estrogen modulation of growth of mouse vaginal epithelium in cell and organ cultures, M.A. thesis in Zoology, University of California, Berkeley (1989).

19. Uchima, F.-D.A., Unpublished.

20. Uchima, F.-D.A., Edery, M., Iguchi, T., Larson, L., and Bern, H.A., Growth of mouse vaginal epithelial cells in culture: Functional integrity of the estrogen receptor system and failure of estrogen to induce proliferation. Cancer Lett., 35:227-235 (1987).

21. Yang, J. and Nandi, S., Growth of cultured cells using collagen as substrate, Inter. Rev. Cytology, 81:249 (1983).

3

Reciprocal Tissue Interactions in Morphogenesis and Hormonal Responsiveness of the Female Reproductive Tract

Robert M. Bigsby
Department of Obstetrics and Gynecology
Indiana University School of Medicine
Indianapolis, Indiana 46223

Summary

A brief review is made of the literature which describes the role of mesenchymal-epithelial interactions in organogenesis of the female reproductive tract and other organs that exhibit developmental sensitivity to steroid hormones. Also reviewed are studies in which the developing neonatal mouse uterus is used as a model for investigating the mechanisms underlying acute effects of estrogen and progesterone on uterine epithelial cell proliferation.

Uterine epithelium of the neonatal Balb/c mouse lacks estrogen receptor, yet, an increase in cellular proliferation occurs when the synthetic estrogen, diethylstilbestrol (DES) is administered to these animals. The presence of estrogen receptors in the mesenchymal cells suggest that this estrogen-induced proliferation may be mediated by mesenchymal factors. Conflicting reports have indicated that epithelial cells of the neonatal mouse uterus do indeed express estrogen receptor, however, upon systematic examination of this issue the apparent discrepancy can be ascribed to developmental differences between the strains of mice used in those studies.

The uterine epithelium of the neonatal mouse exhibits a high rate of cellular proliferation in the absence of steroid hormones. Progesterone inhibition of this proliferative activity is taken to indicate that the mechanism of progesterone action does not require perturbation of estrogen receptor activity. Tissue recombinant studies indicate that there is a mesenchymal component required for the inhibitory activity of progesterone.

In developmental studies and tissue recombinant experiments, it was found that specific cytokeratin peptides are expressed during the early stages of mesenchymally induced cytodifferentiation. It is hoped that this will serve as a marker in further studies designed to elucidate the mechanisms of these tissue interactions.

Introduction

The importance of mesenchymal-epithelial interactions in development is well recognized. During the process of organogenesis the interaction of the two constituent tissues of the primordial organ, the mesenchyme and the epithelium, is crucial for the induction of differentiation and ultimate morphogenesis of the epithelial parenchyma. Experimental studies in which mesenchymal and epithelial components of two organs are separated and recombined in a heterologous fashion have shown that mesenchyme is capable of altering the morphogenetic fate of an epithelium. Examples of this type of instructive induction have been demonstrated for epithelial morphogenesis in such diverse organs as teeth (28), avian cutaneous appendages (47), male accessory sex glands (12, 13), and the female reproductive tract (9, 13). Alternatively, the differentiation of a tissue may not require a specific inducer but rather association with one of any of several tissues will permit a predetermined morphogenesis to occur. The best studied example of such a permissive induction is the differentiation of kidney tubule epithelium (18, 23, 46, 59). Presumably, the signals generated by the inducing tissue can be specific for the responding tissue or they can be of a general nature, allowing the expression of a predetermined phenotype; additionally, the responding tissue may be competent to respond to either specific or general signals. In the mature organ, the connective tissue subjacent to the epithelium is referred to as the stroma, a mesenchymal derivative composed of fibroblastic cells and an abundance of extracellular material. It is likely that stromal-epithelial interactions are also important in the maintenance of structure and function in the mature organ (10). It is hoped that by studying developmental processes, and by using the techniques of developmental biology, we can gain understanding of the mechanisms that are involved in physiologic regulation of mature tissues.

Mesenchymal-epithelial interactions are also known to be crucial to some hormonally dependent developmental processes and it is likely that these interactions are pertinent to the hormonal responsiveness of the fully developed organs as well. Prostatic morphogenesis of the urogenital sinus epithelium requires androgen stimulation. During development, it is the mesenchymal component of the prostatic anlagen that contains androgen receptor and, in experimental tissue recombinations, it has been clearly demonstrated that it is the androgen receptor of the mesenchyme that mediates androgen effects on glandular differentiation (12, 13). Furthermore, in mature prostatic epithelium, androgen-induced epithelial proliferation is dependent upon the stromal androgen receptor (53). In the late stages of fetal lung development, a glucocorticoid-dependent event triggers epithelial production of surfactant. It is the lung mesenchymal cells that directly respond to glucocorticoid by synthesizing and secreting a growth factor which acts upon the epithelium to induce the necessary cytodifferentiation leading to surfactant production (50). Androgens induce degeneration of the mammary epithelium in the males of certain strains of mice; it is the mesenchymal cells surrounding the epithelium that mediate this effect (30). These examples of hormonally dependent responses suggest that mesenchymal-epithelial interactions might exist for other hormonally dependent developmental processes and that such interactions might be carried over as a mechanism of hormone action in mature organs. Indeed, one might expect the mechanisms involved in fetal organ development to be especially relevant in an organ such as the uterus which undergoes cyclic rounds of morphogenesis and atrophy due to the cyclically changing hormonal milieu.

Developmental effects of sex hormones are lasting, leading to sexually dimorphic tissue growth and function that is apparent in adulthood. Studying the permanent malformation or dysfunction induced by application of excess hormone, or hormone withdrawal following ablation of endocrine organs, during development can lead to an understanding of the mechanisms regulating the normal, mature organ. The reproductive tract of the neonatal female mouse can be considered to be developmentally equivalent to that of the human fetus at 15-20 weeks of gestation (2, 21, 22). It is therefore pertinent that the synthetic estrogen, diethylstilbestrol (DES), administered to neonatal mice produces a disruption of the normal mechanisms which control growth of the vaginal epithelium in adulthood, producing such disorders as persistent, ovary-independent, vaginal cornification; hyperplastic lesions; cervicovaginal cancer; and vaginal adenosis (2, 21). The relevance of studying this animal model is emphasized by the occurrence of a similar range of non-neoplastic, preneoplastic, and neoplastic lesions in the vaginae and cervices of women that were exposed to this potent estrogen in utero (49). Results from tissue recombination experiments suggest that the DES-induced permanent perturbation of growth control in the mouse vagina can be attributed to effects of the synthetic hormone on the mesenchyme of the developing organ (14). Again, such observations support the notion that the stroma of the adult organ is an important component of the mechanism controlling growth of a hormonally responsive epithelium. In addition to the developmental aspects, the neonatal mouse offers a unique model for studying acute hormonal responses in uterine tissues. The epithelium of the uterus of the newborn

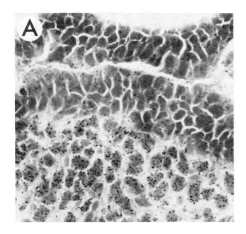
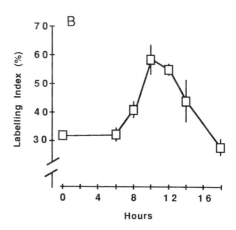

Figure 1. Estradiol Autoradiography and Epithelial Thymidine Labelling Index. A, Uterus of a 4-day-old Balb/c mouse processed for estradiol autoradiography. Notice the lack of silver grain concentration over the nuclei of the epithelial cells. B, Thymidine labelling index (percentage of cells incorporating ^{3}H-TdR) in the epithelium of a 5-day-old Balb/c mouse; ^{3}H-TdR was administered at times indicated after a single dose of the synthetic estrogen, diethylstilbestrol. [from Bigsby & Cunha, 1986 (4), with permission]

mouse lacks estrogen receptor; yet, when estrogen is administered the rate of DNA synthesis and mitotic activity is increased in this tissue (Figure 1). The time course of the epithelial DNA synthetic response shown for neonatal mouse uterus is the same as that observed in the uterus of adult, ovariectomized mouse (37, 38), suggesting that the mechanism is the same in each case. Therefore, it appears that estrogen acts indirectly on the epithelium to induce cellular proliferation. Since the mesenchymal component of the organ is composed of estrogen receptor positive cells, it is likely that it is involved in mediating the hormonal response. Using tissue recombination experiments, Cunha and coworkers (8, 13) have shown that differentiation and morphogenesis of the epithelia of the uterus and vagina are mesenchymally directed; accordingly, uterine epithelium grown on vaginal stroma gives rise to a stratified squamous epithelium that cornifies and keratinizes in response to estrogen, while vaginal epithelium grown on uterine stroma yields a columnar epithelium, the height of which is under estrogen control. Thus, as in other developing organ systems, the mesenchyme of the uterus governs epithelial growth and differentiation; in the mature uterus, the processes governing epithelial proliferation and morphogenesis are directed by ovarian steroids. Implicit in this statement is the notion that it is the interaction of epithelium with its mesenchyme, or stroma, that comes under the control of ovarian hormones.

Insight into the mechanisms by which progesterone inhibits estrogen-induced proliferation of uterine epithelial cells can also be gained through studies of the neonatal mouse uterus. It is generally held that progesterone blocks estrogen induction of uterine growth by perturbing the mechanisms by which estrogen acts. That is, progesterone inhibits synthesis of estrogen receptor (24), particularly that of the epithelium in the uterus (45, 55); and decreases binding of estrogen receptor to its nuclear accepter (32, 44). The obvious conclusion to be drawn from this information is that by inhibiting the mechanisms through which estrogen acts, progesterone inhibits estrogen induction of uterine epithelial proliferation. However, results derived from studies on the neonatal mouse bring this conclusion into question. During the first two weeks after birth, the rate of DNA synthesis is high in both the mesenchyme and the epithelium of the uterus and remains so after ovariectomy and adrenalectomy, suggesting that the cells of the uterus are proliferating independently of estrogen (43). Yet when progesterone is administered, the DNA synthetic and mitotic activities of the epithelium are specifically inhibited (Figure 2; cf. 6).

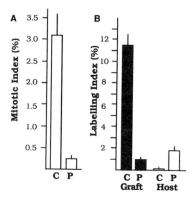

Figure 2. Progesterone Inhibition of Estrogen-Independent Proliferation in Neonatal Mouse Uterine Epithelium. A, Mitotic index of the uterine epithelium was determined following a single injection of progesterone to 4-day-old Balb/c mice. At 24 h after progesterone treatment, colchicine was administered to each of 5 animals per group and 2 h later the reproductive tracts were removed. The number of cells arrested in mitosis was related to the total of at least 1000 cells counted. Mitotic index of the progesterone-treated group (P) was significantly reduced compared to vehicle-treated controls (C). B, Thymidine labelling index was determined for the epithelium of neonatal mouse uterine pieces grown as grafts in ovariectomized, adult hosts. Uterine pieces from 1-day-old Balb/c mice were grafted under the kidney capsules of syngeneic adults that had been ovariectomized 6 weeks earlier. The epithelial labelling indices of grafted tissue and of the host's uterus was determined 9 days later, 18 h after an injection of progesterone (P, 40 μg/g BW) or its vehicle (C, sesame oil). The host epithelium was nearly devoid of any thymidine labelling, indicating a lack of any uterotrophic estrogen, yet the grafted tissue exhibited a relatively high index that was decreased by progesterone treatment. [from Bigsby & Cunha, 1985 (3), with permission].

This suggests that progesterone does not act on this aspect of uterine epithelial physiology by perturbation of the mechanisms of estrogen action; it is quite possible that decreased estrogen receptor content and activity are merely coincident with, not causal to, blockade of estrogen induction of mitosis. This idea is further supported by the observation that progesterone inhibits epithelial DNA synthesis in another model of estrogen-independent uterine growth. Cholera toxin introduced into the lumen of ovariectomized rats causes a true growth response without activating the estrogen receptor system (52, 60). When the animals are pretreated with progesterone the epithelial response to cholera toxin is blocked (Table 1). Disruption of estrogen receptor activity is therefore not a prerequisite for progestin inhibition of uterine epithelial proliferation, it is more likely that progestin action results in the coincidental down regulation of a number of cellular activities including estrogen receptor synthesis, nuclear estrogen receptor binding, and DNA synthesis. We must reexamine this problem, searching for alternative mechanisms that explain these new observations. The possibility that the uterine stroma plays a role in mediating the inhibitory action of progesterone is examined in experiments described below.

Not only does the mesenchyme influence morphogenesis and hormonal responsiveness of the epithelium but so too does the epithelium affect the mesenchymal component of the organ. During development, the uterine mesenchyme gives rise to the myometrium and endometrial stroma. Cunha (16) has recently shown that differentiation of myometrial tissue within the developing mesenchyme is dependent upon an intact epithelium. Mature uterine stroma also exhibits a requirement for the effect of its overlying epithelium. In progesterone-treated, ovariectomized rats, traumatization of the uterine tissues leads to growth of the stromal compartment (33). This decidualization reaction can be elicited by passing suture thread through the uterine wall, scratching the luminal surface, or by momentarily crushing the tissues with a pair of forceps. This stromal growth response is absent if the epithelium has been ablated (33, 34). Thus, communication across the basement membrane is not unidirectional.

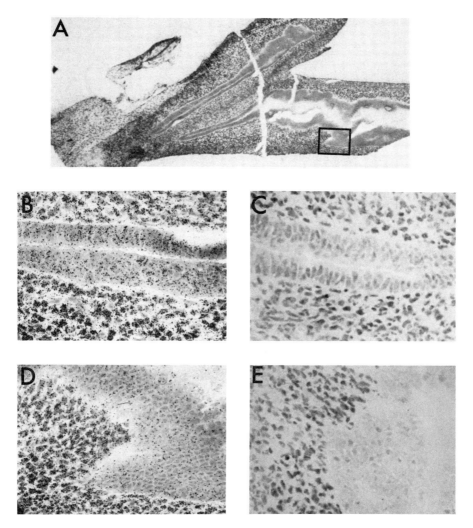

Figure 3. Comparison of Estradiol Autoradiography and Estrogen Receptor Immunocytochemistry. The reproductive tract of a 5-day-old CD-1 mouse was incubated in ^{3}H-estradiol, frozen and sectioned. Alternate longitudinal sections were thaw-mounted on emulsion-coated slides for autoradiography and on lysine-coated slides for immunocytochemistry. A. Low magnification showing a longitudinal section containing the middle and lower (cervical end) regions of the uterine horns; boxes indicate the regions of the lower uterus and the middle uterus that are examined at higher magnification: B & C, lower uterus; D & E, middle uterus. Estradiol autoradiography (B & D) clearly show that there are more estrogen receptor positive epithelial cells in the lower uterus and that those cells that are positive in the middle uterus have fewer silver grains below their nuclei than those of the lower uterus. Immunocytochemistry yields a similar result, the number and intensity of positive epithelial cells being greater in the lower uterus (C & E) [from Bigsby *et al*, 1990 (5), with permission].

As mentioned above, the lack of estrogen receptor in the uterine epithelium of the neonatal mouse has lead to the hypothesis that there is a mesenchymal component required for estrogen-induced cellular proliferation in that tissue. However, Korach (29) has published immunocytochemical evidence that some of the epithelial cells in the uterus of neonatal mice do exhibit estrogen receptor protein (29, 61). As reported in a preliminary study, reconciliation of this apparent discrepancy lies in the fact that there are developmental differences between the different strains of mice used in each of these studies (5); further systematic examination of this topic is described in the present studies.

Tissue recombinant experiments are also described which examine the role of the uterine stroma in progesterone blockade of estrogen-induced epithelial proliferation. These studies take advantage of the fact that progesterone blocks estrogen-induced epithelial proliferation in the uterus but not in the vagina (31). Additionally, epithelial cytokeratin expression during stromally induced epithelial differentiation is examined and results suggest that these cytoskeletal proteins may act as an early marker of such differentiation.

Materials and Methods

Postnatal Expression of Estrogen Receptor in the Murine Uterus

The reproductive tracts of neonatal females of an inbred strain of mice, Balb/c and the outbred strain, CD-1 were used. Pregnant females were housed in a controlled environment with a 12 hour light period commencing at 6 AM. Each morning and afternoon cages were examined for the presence of pups. Tracts were collected from animals that were 1- to 9-days-old. The cellular content of estrogen receptor was examined in the tissues of these tracts using estradiol autoradiography and/or immunocytochemistry. One group of Balb/c mice was treated with DES (1 μg/10 μl sesame seed oil, ip) in the evening when they were 2-days-old and 14 h later, when they were 3-days-old, their tracts were collected for estrogen receptor immunocytochemistry.

Immunostaining of estrogen receptor was performed using the monoclonal antibody, H222, developed by G. Greene and supplied by Abbott Laboratories (Arlington Heights, IL). As in the study of Yamashita and Korach (61) the tissues to be analyzed were fixed in buffered formalin at 4°C for 60-90 min., washed overnight at 4°C in phosphate buffered saline (PBS) containing 7.5% sucrose. Entire tracts were embedded in HistoPrep embedding medium (Fisher, Itasca, IL), frozen in liquified propane that was maintained at liquid nitrogen temperature, and stored submersed in liquid nitrogen until sectioning. Four micron longitudinal sections were thaw mounted onto lysine-coated slides and held at -20°C in storage medium (equal volumes of glycerol and PBS containing 0.5 M sucrose, 14 mM MgCl$_2$) until immunostained. Following incubation in normal sheep serum (1% in PBS) to block nonspecific antibody binding, the sections were incubated in H222. The anti-estrogen receptor antibody was visualized using a biotinylated anti-rat Ig (Amersham Research Products, Arlington Heights, IL) and the avidin, biotinylated peroxidase system (Vector Labs, Burlingame, CA) with diaminobenzidine/H$_2$O$_2$ (Sigma Chemicals, St. Louis, MO) as the substrate solution. (Best delineation between immuno-positive nuclei and immuno-negative nuclei was obtained when the sections were also stained lightly with hematoxylin; however, this procedure was omitted so that the reader could make that delineation while viewing the black and white photomicrographs presented herein.)

Estrogen receptor autoradiography was performed as described earlier (4). Briefly, the reproductive tracts were incubated for 1 h at 37°C in Ham's F12 nutrient mixture containing 0.05% bovine serum albumin (BSA) and 10 nM ^{3}H-estradiol. The tissue samples were then washed in 6 changes of phosphate buffered saline containing 0.05% BSA at 4°C over a 3 h period. Tissue was then embedded in HistoPrep and frozen in liquid propane as above. Frozen sections (4 μm) were thaw-mounted onto slides previously coated with photographic emulsion (NTB-2, Kodak, Rochester, NY). After 8 weeks exposure at -70°C, the slides were developed (D-19, Kodak), fixed, and stained with hematoxylin and eosin.

Tissue Recombinants and Progesterone Inhibition of Epithelial DNA Synthesis

Epithelium and mesenchyme of the vagina and the uterus from neonatal (0 - 2 days of age) Fisher 344 rats (Harlan, Indianapolis) were separated enzymatically and recombined in a heterologous fashion. Heterotypic tissue recombinants were made: vaginal mesenchyme plus uterine epithelium (VgM + UtE), and the converse, uterine mesenchyme plus vaginal epithelium (UtM + VgE). Homotypic recombinants (VgM + VgE; UtM + UtE) were also made as controls. These tissue recombinants were incubated overnight on agar coated dishes

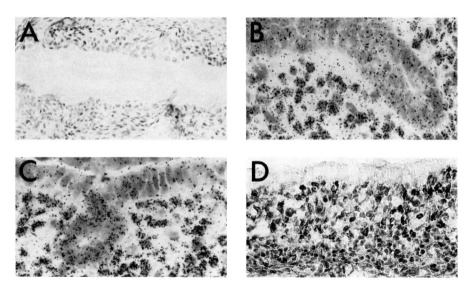

Figure 4. Comparison of Estrogen Receptor Ontogeny in Different Strains of Mice. A, Immunocytochemistry of estrogen receptor in the uterus of a 2-day-old CD-1 mouse. B, & C, Estradiol autoradiography of the uteri from a 4-day-old CD-1 mouse (B), a 5-day-old CD-1 mouse (C). D, Estrogen receptor immunocytochemistry of the uterus from a 6-day-old Balb/c mouse.

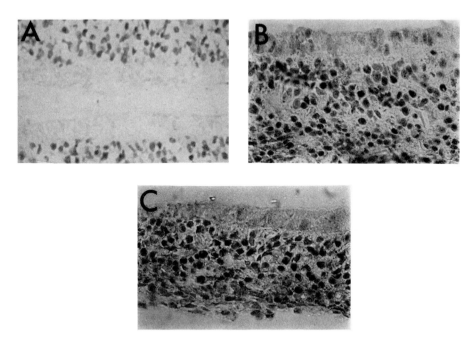

Figure 5. Estrogen Receptor Immunocytochemistry and Thymidine Autoradiography following Estrogen Stimulation. Reproductive tracts were collected from Balb/c mice that were 3 or 5 days-old and that had been treated with DES 14 h earlier. Epithelium of a uterus from a 3-day-old animal is devoid of receptor immunostaining (A). Epithelium of the lower uterus (B) of a 5-day-old animal shows numerous positive cells, while in the middle region of the same uterus (C) only a few cells are positive.

Table 1. Effect of Progesterone on Cholera Toxin Stimulation of Uterine Epithelial Growth. Cholera toxin (50 μl, 0.4 μg/ml) was injected into the uterine lumens of ovariectomized rats. Twenty hours later, ^{3}H-TdR was administered ip. Thymidine labelling index and cell height were determined in luminal epithelium of uterine specimens taken from animals that had been treated with sesame oil (vehicle), or progesterone prior to intraluminal cholera toxin (CT) injection or sham injection [from Bigsby & Cunha, 1988 (6), with permission]

Treatment			Epithelial Response	
Animal	Intraut	(n)	Labelling (%)	Height (μm)
Vehicle	Sham	(3)	0.53 ± 0.15	10.5 ± 1.14
Progest	Sham	(4)	0.00 ± 0.00	12.0 ± 0.19
Vehicle	CT	(6)	5.20 ± 1.10	24.8 ± 2.12
Progest	CT	(6)	0.15 ± 0.08	13.0 ± 0.66

as described earlier (9). Tissue recombinants were then grown under the kidney capsules of adult, syngeneic female rats. Additional pieces of mesenchyme that were not recombined with epithelium were grafted as controls; if histological examination of these showed epithelial contamination then the group of recombinants made with that mesenchyme was disregarded. After one month, the hosts were ovariectomized and one week later they were treated with two daily doses of progesterone (40 μg/g BW, sc) or its vehicle (Moleculsol, Pharmatec Co., Alachua, FL). One hour after the second dose of progesterone, hosts received an injection of estradiol (1.25 μg, sc) or its vehicle (sesame oil). Twenty hours later each host received an ip injection of ^{3}H-thymidine (^{3}H-TdR, 1.5 μCi/g BW). After an additional hour, the animals were killed. Both the host's reproductive tract and the recombinants were placed in neutral formalin and processed for paraffin embedding. Six micron sections were mounted on BSA coated slides; the slides were dehydrated, dried and dipped in photographic emulsion. After a 4 week exposure at -70°C, slides were developed as above and stained with hematoxylin and eosin.

Another set of tissue recombinants was made with mesenchyme from neonatal vagina (VgM$_2$) or uterus (UtM$_2$) and epithelium from uterus of 10- to 16-day-old Fisher 344 rats (UtE$_{10}$). These heterochronal recombinants (VgM$_2$ + UtE$_{10}$; UtM$_2$ + UtE$_{10}$) were grown under the renal capsules of syngeneic female hosts. The hosts were ovariectomized, treated with steroids and ^{3}H-TdR, as above. The host's tract and the grafted tissues were processed for autoradiography.

Developmental Expression of Cytokeratin Peptides

Reproductive tracts were removed from neonatal Fisher 344 rats at ages 1- through 6-days, at 20-days and 60-days. The tissues were embedded in HistoPrep and frozen in liquified propane. Frozen sections (4 μm) were thaw mounted onto lysine-coated slides. Sections were stained with the following anti-cytokeratin monoclonal antibodies: AE8 (a gift from Dr. T-T Sun, New York University), PKK1 (Labsystems, Helsinki), K8.12, or K4.62 (ICN Immunobiologicals, Lisle, IL). The mouse monoclonal antibodies were detected with the ABC Vectastain^c (Vector Labs) kit using diaminobenzidine as the substrate.

Tissue recombinants VgM + UtE, were from organs of neonatal rats. These were grafted and grown as above, except they were removed from hosts after 1 week. Experience (unpublished) had shown that mesenchymal induction of the epithelium was incomplete at this point, some of the epithelium was still simple, columnar, while some epithelium had already undergone full transformation into the stratified, squamous histotype. Thus, the epithelium could be studied during differentiation as directed by the mesenchyme. These week-old grafts were frozen, sectioned and processed for cytokeratin immunohistochemistry.

Table 2. Cytokeratin Antibodies and Predicted Immunostaining. The monoclonal antibodies used in the immunohistochemical analyses are listed. The human cytokeratin proteins with which they react, according to their molecular weight and the numbering system of Moll (40), is also listed. The predicted cell type which these antibodies will react is derived from the categorization of the numbered cytokeratins according to by Sun (54)

Antibody	Predicted Epithelial Staining (Cytokeratin Reactive)	Simple	Stratified
PKK1	52k(8), 48k(?) 45k(18), 40k(19)	+	--
K4.62	40k(19)	+	--
K8.12	51k(13), 48k(16)	--	+
K8.6	68k(1), 56.5k(10), 56k(11)	--	+
AE8	51k(13)	--	+

Results

Postnatal Expression of Estrogen Receptor

It has been suggested (29, 61) that immunocytochemical analysis of estrogen receptor is more sensitive than the autoradiographic techniques used in a previous study (4). When the two techniques are compared directly on serial sections of the same tissue it is apparent that no such discrepancy exists (Figure 3). Indeed, the uterine epithelium of the 5-day-old CD-1 mouse exhibits a positional gradient of estrogen receptor expression, the caudal uterus (Figure 3b & c) having more positive cells with greater intensity of labelling than the more cephalic regions (Figure 3d & e). This pattern has been observed in the other strains of mice examined, except that the age at which the epithelium begins to express the receptor varies. To illustrate the differences in the strains of mice in this regard, Figure 4A shows that the uterine epithelium of a 2-day-old CD-1 mouse is estrogen receptor negative while that of a 4-day-old CD-1 mouse (Figure 4B) has a number of positive cells. In the uterus of a 5-day-old CD-1 mouse there is an epithelial structure which resembles a gland; the cells of this structure exhibit a more intense concentration of the radiolabelled steroid than the other epithelial cells (Figure 4C) The epithelium of a 6-day-old Balb/c mouse is devoid of estrogen receptor (Figure 4D). The apparent glandular budding of the epithelium of the 5-day-old CD-1 mouse is a further manifestation of the advanced maturity of the epithelium of that strain compared to the inbred Balb/c animals; in the latter strain no such epithelial structures were evident until 7-days of age. Clearly, although there are strain dependent differences in the age at which estrogen receptor first appears in the uterine epithelium, there is no discrepancy between the autoradiographic data and the immunocytochemical data.

The conclusion drawn from an earlier study (4) was that the epithelium of the neonatal mouse (4- to 5-day-old Balb/c) responded to estrogen stimulation even though its cells were devoid of estrogen receptor. Since the 5-day-old Balb/c mouse is close to the developmental stage at which the uterine epithelial cells express estrogen receptor, this experiment was repeated using 2-day-old animals; again, the epithelial thymidine labelling index was nearly doubled by DES treatment (56). In the present investigation, the uteri of similarly treated 2- and 4-day-old Balb/c mice were examined for estrogen receptor immunostaining before and after treatment. The epithelium of the younger animals remained devoid of estrogen receptor 14 hours following DES treatment (Figure 5A), while in some of the 5-day-old, DES-treated animals, epithelium showed precocious expression of estrogen receptor, particularly in the lower uterus (Figures 5B & C). Thus, although estrogen treatment induces early expression of estrogen receptor, this is not a prerequisite to estrogen-induced epithelial DNA synthesis.

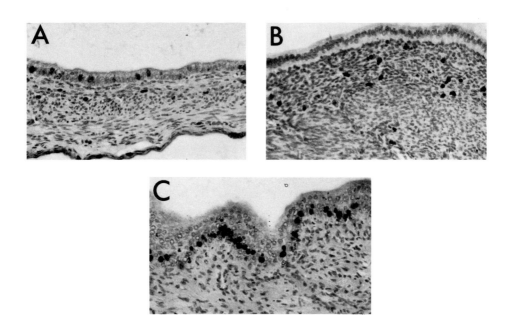

Figure 6. Effect of Combined Progesterone and Estradiol treatment on DNA Synthesis in Heterotypic Tissue Recombinants. Heterotypic tissue recombinants were made from tissues of neonatal rats. Vaginal and uterine tissues were separated and recombined in a heterologous manner. Autoradiographs of UtM + VgE show intense thymidine labelling of the columnar epithelium following treatment of the host with estradiol alone (A) and the lack of labelling in the epithelium following combined progesterone and estradiol treatment (B). Estrogen also induces DNA synthetic activity in the basal epithelial layer of VgM + UtE recombinants; this estrogen response is not blocked in the epithelium by progesterone treatment (C).

Progesterone Inhibition of Epithelial DNA Synthesis

In the ovariectomized rat, estrogen stimulates proliferation of the epithelia of both the uterus and the vagina; progesterone blocks this estrogen effect in the uterus only (31). These observations were used to test the hypothesis that there is a stromal component to the mechanisms by which progesterone blocks uterine epithelial proliferation.

Morphogenesis and hormonal responsiveness of uterine epithelium of neonatal (0- to 2-days-old) rats (UtE$_2$) recombined with mesenchyme of neonatal vagina or uterus proceed along the path directed by the mesenchyme. That is, UtE$_2$ grown on uterine mesenchyme remains columnar, is stimulated by estrogen, and estrogen stimulation of growth is blocked by progesterone; whereas, UtE$_2$ grown on vaginal mesenchyme becomes stratified, proliferates in response to estrogen, but is not inhibited by progesterone (Fig. 6).

When uterine epithelium from a neonatal mouse is recombined with neonatal vaginal mesenchyme the epithelium becomes stratified (as shown above), however, when the epithelium is derived from the uterus of an animal that is 10-days-old, or older, it does not undergo the morphologic transformation into a stratified phenotype (unpublished). The older epithelium is apparently fully determined so that it remains as uterine epithelium when grown on this foreign mesenchyme. The altered hormonal responsiveness of the neonatal uterine epithelium grown on vaginal mesenchyme may be a result of the altered cytoarchitecture following stratification and can be considered as an indication of the completeness of mesenchymally induced vaginal morphogenesis. By using the older epithelium in tissue recombinant experiments, hormonal responsiveness can be tested in the absence of these dramatic morphogenetic changes. Figure 7 shows that proliferation of the

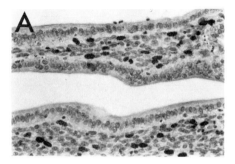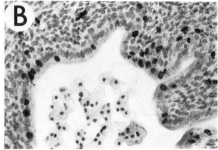

Figure 7. Effect of Combined Progesterone and Estradiol Treatment on DNA Synthesis in Heterochronal Tissue Recombinants. Uterine epithelium from 10- to 16-day-old rats (UtE_{10}) remains columnar when grown on uterine or vaginal mesenchyme from 0- to 2-day-old rats (UtM_2 and VgM_2, respectively). When the hosts were treated with a combination of progesterone plus estradiol, thymidine labelling of the epithelium was blocked in the UtM_2 + UtE_{10} recombinants (A) while labelling of the epithelium in the VgM_2 + UtE_{10} recombinants was not blocked (B).

epithelium of tissue recombinants made using 10-day-old uterine epithelium (UtE_{10}) is inhibited by progesterone when it is grown on uterine mesenchyme (UtM_2 + UtE_{10}, epithelial labelling index: 0.7±0.4%, n = 3, mean ± SEM) but its proliferation is unaffected by progesterone when it is associated with vaginal mesenchyme (VgM_2 + UtE_{10}, epithelial labelling index\: 12.6 ± 2.4%, n = 3, mean ± SEM). Thus, even though the UtE_{10} retained its morphologic characteristics it responded to progesterone only when it was associated with uterine mesenchyme. These results are consistent with the concept of a progesterone-sensitive factor produced by the uterine stroma, but not the vaginal stroma, that acts on uterine epithelium to inhibit cell proliferation.

Developmental Expression of Cytokeratin Peptides

As shown above epithelial morphogenesis is directed by the mesenchyme with which it is associated. In the case of vaginal mesenchyme, the overlying epithelium is induced to form a stratified histotype. Intuitively, one would expect that an early event in the transformation of a columnar epithelium into stratified epithelial architecture might be the restructuring of the cytoarchitecture of the cells involved. The intermediate filaments of the epithelial cell cytoskeleton are composed of pairs of a family of proteins known as cytokeratins. The 20+ cytokeratins known to exist in a given species can be categorized as to the type of epithelium in which they are found (54); accordingly, there are cytokeratins of simple epithelia (all cells maintain contact with the basement membrane) which are distinct from those found in stratified epithelia (only the basal layer of cells maintain direct contact with the basement membrane). If transformation of the cytoarchitecture is an early event in the transformation of the histoarchitecture, then expression of specific cytokeratins representative of the new phenotype may occur early in this process. This possibility was examined in normally developing rat reproductive tracts and in tissue recombinant studies.

The battery of monoclonal antibodies used in the following studies were chosen because the proteins with which they react have been categorized as occurring in either stratified or simple epithelia. The antibodies and the immunocytochemical staining predicted from their known reactivities are summarized in Table 2. The stratified epithelia of the vagina and cervix and the simple epithelium of the uterus in the adult rat exhibit the predicted immunostaining. Figures 8A & B show examples of the immunostaining of adult uterus and vagina. The epithelia of the upper vagina and cervix of the neonatal (0 - 4 days old) rat are simple (21, 22). These epithelia stain with anti-cytokeratin antibodies against both simple-

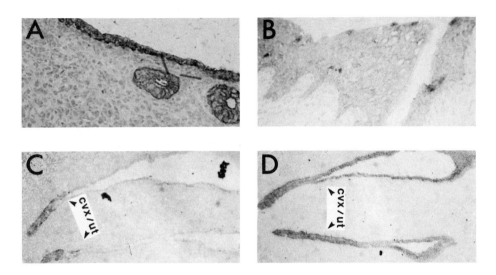

Figure 8. Cytokeratin Expression in Reproductive Tract Development. Adult rat uterus was stained with PKK1 (A) and vagina with K8.12 (B). Adjacent longitudinal sections of neonatal (3-day-old) rat tracts were stained with K8.12 (C) and K4.62 (D); the same region of epithelium is designated as the cervical-uterine junction (cvx/ut) in these sections.

type and stratified-type cytokeratin proteins, as exemplified in Figures 8C & D. Thus, in normal development of the lower reproductive tract, the transformation of the simple epithelium into a stratified epithelium is preceded by expression of the cytokeratin proteins of the stratified-type cell.

Tissue recombinants made of neonatal VgM and UtE yield a fully stratified epithelium after 4 weeks growth in an intact female host. If the grafts are harvested early, after 1 week of growth, the epithelium is only partially transformed into a stratified phenotype, i.e., some simple, columnar epithelium may be found within the recombinant (unpublished). When this experiment was performed, the simple epithelium found in the VgM + UtE tissue recombinant stained with the monospecific monoclonal antibody, AE8, which recognizes a cytokeratin protein found only in stratified epithelia (Figure 9B). The stratified epithelium that was present stained with all three antibodies against stratified-type cytokeratins (as in Figure 9A). These observations suggest that specific cytokeratin expression is one of the early events in mesenchymally induced epithelial stratification.

Discussion

When examined systematically using both immunocytochemical techniques and steroid autoradiography, it is apparent that the estrogen receptor system of uterine epithelium in the outbred strain, CD-1, used by Korach (29, 61) for their studies, develops at a rate that is 2-3 days ahead of either of two inbred strains, Balb/c (present study) or C57Bl/6J (56). Moreover, the earlier onset of epithelial maturation is also seen in CD-1 mice when uterine glandular morphogenesis is used as the criterion. Additionally, Andersson and Forsberg (1) found that the uterine epithelium of neonatal (0- to 5-days-old) NMRI mice did not exhibit immunostaining with the anti-estrogen receptor antibody. Differences among strains of mice with regard to development and hormonal sensitivity have long been known (7, 37, 41). This being the case, it appears that the conclusion drawn earlier still holds, i.e., uterine epithelial estrogen receptor is not required for estrogen induction of cellular proliferation in that tissue of neonatal mice (4, 56). And again, the similarity of the time course of estrogen

22

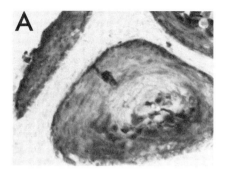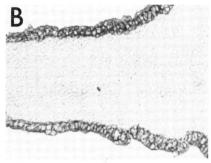

Figure 9. Cytokeratin Expression in VgM + UtE Tissue Recombinants. Tissue recombinants, VgM + UtE, were harvested after 1 week of growth in a syngeneic host. Some of the epithelium developed into a fully stratified phenotype and this stained with all three stratified-type cytokeratin antibodies, K8.12 staining is shown (A). Other epithelial cells in the same tissue recombinant had not undergone stratification, yet they stained with AE8(B).

stimulation in the uterus of the neonatal mouse (Figure 1) and in the uterus of the adult animal (38) suggests that the mechanism is the same in both. Since the mesenchymal, or stromal, cells of these uteri express estrogen receptor, they may also mediate the hormonal response.

Analogy to the mesenchymally directed epithelial morphogenesis in the female reproductive tract argues for a role of the mesenchyme, or stroma, in estrogen-induced epithelial growth. Nonetheless, estrogen-induced proliferation in the epithelia of heterotypic tissue recombinants does not indicate an active role of the stroma in mediating estrogen responsiveness. However, experiments with uterine cells in culture do support the notion of an active stromal mediation. In numerous reported attempts, estrogen failed to stimulate proliferation of isolated uterine or vaginal epithelia in cell culture (21, 25, 27, 35, 57). On the other hand, when cultured vaginal or uterine epithelial cells were reassociated with their respective stroma and grown as subcapsular renal grafts, estrogen stimulated cell proliferation (8). Estrogen also stimulated uterine epithelial cells that remained associated with their stroma in organ culture (39) or that were grown in cell culture admixed with stromal cells (26). Such observations further support the hypothesis that stroma mediates the proliferative effect of estrogen.

Cellular proliferation is one of the early steps in the process of tissue morphogenesis. Estrogen receptor expression in the uterine epithelial cell can be considered an indication of the progressive cytodifferentiation required to reach full morphogenesis and function of the tissue. Thus, those epithelial cells that stain for estrogen receptor in the uterus of 5-day-old Balb/c mice that had been treated with DES have been induced to differentiate prematurely. Andersson and Forsberg (1) reported a similar finding in neonatal NMRI mice; they also reported that 5 days of estrogen treatment induced precocious morphogenesis of a stratified epithelium in the vagina of this strain. Both the basal and superficial cells of this newly stratified epithelium were positive for estrogen receptor immunostaining; the authors argue that since the superficial cells were not in contact with the basement membrane, their expression of estrogen receptor could not be due to a stromal factor. Taguchi (56) had reported that 3 days of prenatal DES treatment induced hyperplasia and precocious expression of estrogen receptor in the vaginal epithelium of C57BL/6J mice but no premature stratification was noted. These results suggest that estrogen induces both proliferation and estrogen receptor expression in the epithelium prior to induction of stratification. The suprabasal layers of a stratified epithelium are formed when the basal cells migrate upward; therefore, the cells occupying the superficial layer in the prematurely stratified vaginal epithelium, as described by Andersson and Forsberg (1), would have been in contact with the basement membrane at the time of estrogen-induced expression of estrogen receptor.

It is thus apparent from the above discussion that, in the female reproductive tract, administration of estrogen can induce early cytodifferentiation and morphogenesis of the epithelia, processes known to be directed by the mesenchyme. It therefore appears likely that estrogen is capable of enhancing mesenchymal signals that regulate epithelial processes. Numerous growth factors have been shown to stimulate epithelial cell proliferation and differentiation, making them candidates for the role of mediating mesenchymal-epithelial interactions. Insulin-like growth factors and epidermal growth factor have been identified as possible paracrine mediators of estrogen-induced growth in the uterus (17, 39, 42, 51); however, these growth factors are not likely to be specific mediators of a stromally induced epithelial response because they either lack tissue specificity or are not derived solely from the stromal compartment. In general, these same reservations apply to most of the other known growth factors when considering them as possible mediators of mesenchymally regulated epithelial growth. However, Finch (19) has recently described a keratinocyte growth factor (KGF) that is produced only in cells of mesenchymal origin and which induces proliferation of only epithelial cells. Whether uterine or vaginal stroma produces KGF, or an equivalent, is yet to be determined.

Data presented here support the idea that there is a stromal component to the mechanism by which progesterone inhibits the uterine epithelium. The observations that progesterone will inhibit cellular proliferation in uterine epithelium which is growing in the absence of estrogenic stimulation (3, 6) strongly argues against the proposition that the mechanism of progesterone's inhibitory action is the perturbation of the estrogen receptor system. It is likely that progesterone acts in a more direct manner, perhaps by stimulating the production of a growth inhibitory factor that acts specifically on the uterine cells. Transforming growth factor-β (TGF-β), a peptide known for its growth inhibitory action, has been found in the uterus of mice, localized within the stroma subjacent to glandular epithelium (57; Anita Roberts, personal communication). Analyses are under way to determine whether progesterone stimulates expression of TGF-β in the mouse uterus.

Cytokeratin peptides may prove helpful in further investigations of mesenchymal-epithelial interactions. Because of technical restrictions, it has not been possible to induce full morphogenesis in culture systems. This is not to say that the inductive process does not occur, but rather, use of morphogenesis may be ill-suited as the experimental endpoint for *in vitro* studies of that process. If cytokeratin expression is an early event in the process perhaps it can be used to discern an effect of mesenchyme on epithelium of a tissue recombinant grown in culture. Sawyer and coworkers (47) have successfully examined mesenchymal-epithelial interactions of developing avian dermal appendages in a chorioallantoic membrane culture system using specific keratin expression as an indication of the inductive process. It is hoped that cytokeratin expression in short term organ cultures of VgM + UtE can be used in a like manner.

In summary, developmental studies and tissue recombinant experiments indicate a role for stromal-epithelial interactions in estrogen and progesterone regulation of uterine cell growth. These interactions may have characteristics of both instructive and permissive inductions. Estrogen stimulation may be mediated by a factor common to both uterine and vaginal mesenchymal cells since the epithelia of the two heterotypic recombinants , VgM + UtE and UtM + VgE, responded and since the epithelia of each of these organs have been shown to be responsive to hormone treatment while lacking in estrogen receptors (cf. 1, 4, 56). Cell and organ culture studies cited from the literature suggest an active role of the uterine stroma in estrogen-induced epithelial proliferation but the specificity of this stromal requirement has not been tested. The stromal component of progesterone's inhibitory action appears to be specific to the uterus. Furthermore, developmental studies (16) and experimental manipulation of adult organs (33, 34) indicate that the tissue interactions within the uterus are reciprocal, i.e., epithelium may be involved in the hormonal regulation of the stroma as well.

Acknowledgments

This work was supported by NIH through grant no. HD23244. The helpful comments of Dr. P. S. Cooke were greatly appreciated.

References

1. Andersson, C. and Forsberg, J.-G., Induction of estrogen receptor, peroxidase activity, and epithelial abnormalities in the mouse uterovaginal epithelium after neonatal treatment with diethylstilbestrol, Teratogen. Carcinogen. Mutagen. 8:347 (1988).
2. Bern, H. A. and Talamantes, F. J., Neonatal mouse models and their relation to disease in the human female, In: *Developmental Effects of Diethylstilbestrol (DES) in Pregnancy*, A. L. Herbst, H. A. Bern, (eds)., New York, Thieme-Stratton, pp. 129-147 (1981).
3. Bigsby, R. M. and Cunha, G. R., Progestin and glucocorticoid inhibition of DNA synthesis in uterine epithelium of the neonatal mouse, Endocrinology 117:2520 (1985).
4. Bigsby, R. M. and Cunha, G. R., Estrogen stimulation of DNA synthesis in epithelium which lacks estrogen receptor, Endocrinology 119:390 (1986).
5. Bigsby, R. M., Li, Aixin, L., Luo, K., and Cunha, G. R., Strain differences in the ontogeny of estrogen receptors in murine uterine epithelium, Endocrinology, *in press*, 1990.
6. Bigsby, R. M. and Cunha, G. R., Progesterone and dexamethasone inhibition of uterine epithelial proliferation in two model systems of estrogen-independent uterine growth, Am. J. Obstet. Gynecol. 158:646 (1988).
7. Chai, C. K. and Dickie, M. M., Endocrine Variations, In: E. L. Green (ed.) *Biology of the Laboratory Mouse*, New York, McGraw-Hill pp.387-403 (1966).
8. Cooke, P.S., Uchima, F.-D. A., Fujii, D. K., Bern, H.A., and Cunha G. R., Restoration of normal morphology and estrogen responsiveness in cultured vaginal and uterine epithelia transplanted with stroma, Proc. Natl. Acad. Sci. USA 83:2109 (1986).
9. Cunha, G. R., Stromal induction and specification of morphogenesis and cytodifferentiation of the epithelia of the Mullerian ducts and urogenital sinus during development of the uterus and vagina in mice, J. Exp. Zool. 196:361 (1976).
10. Cunha, G. R., Bigsby, R. M., Cooke, P. S. and Sugimura, Y., Stromal-epithelial interactions in adult organs, Cell Differentiation 17:137 (1985).
11. Cunha, G. R., Bigsby, R. M., Cooke, P. S., and Sugimura, Y., Stromal-epithelial interactions in the determination of hormone responsiveness, In: *Estrogens in the Environment II*, J.A. McLachlan, (ed.) Elsevier, New York, pp. 273-287 (1985).
12. Cunha, G. R. and Chung, L. W. K., Stromal-epithelial interactions: Induction of prostatic phenotype in urothelium of testicular feminized (Tfm/y) mice, J. Steroid Biochem. 14:1317 (1981).
13. Cunha, G. R., Chung, L. W. K., Shannon, J. M., Taguchi, O., and Fujii, H., Hormone-induced morphogenesis and growth: Role of mesenchymal epithelial interactions, Rec. Prog. Horm. Res. 39:559 (1983).
14. Cunha, G. R., Lung, G., and Kato, K., Role of the epithelial-stromal interaction during the development and expression of ovary-independent vaginal hyperplasia, Develop. Biol. 56:52 (1977).
15. Cunha, G. R. and Vanderslice, K. D., Identification in histological sections of species origin of cells from mouse, rat and human, Stain Tech. 59:712 (1984).
16. Cunha, G. R., Young, P., and Brody, J. R., Role of uterine epithelium in the development of myometrial smooth muscle cells, Biol. Reprod. 40:861 (1989).
17. DiAugustine, R. P., Petrusz P., Bell, G. I., Brown, C. F., Korach, K., S., McLachlan, J. A., and Teng, C. T., Influence of estrogens on mouse uterine epidermal growth factor precursor protein and messenger ribonucleic acid, Endocrinology 122:2355 (1988).
18. Ekblom, P., Basement membrane proteins and growth factors in kidney differentiation, In: R.L. Trelstad, (ed.) *The Role of Extracellular Matrix in Development*, Alan R. Liss, New York, pp. 173-206 (1984).

19. Finch, P. W., Rubin, J. S., Miki, T., Ron, D., and Aaronson, S. A. Human KGF is FGF-related with properties of a paracrine effector of epithelial cell growth, Sci. 245:752 (1989).

20. Flaxman, B. A., Chopra, D. P., and Newman, D., Growth of mouse vaginal epithelial cells *in vitro, In Vitro* 9:194 (1973).

21. Forsberg, J.-G. and Kalland, T., Neonatal estrogen treatment and epithelial abnormalities in the cervicovaginal epithelium of adult mice, Cancer Res. 41:721 (1981).

22. Forsberg, J.-G. and Kalland, T., Embryology of the genital tract in humans and in rodents, In: A. L. Herbst, H. A. Bern,(eds.), *Developmental Effects of Diethylstilbestrol (DES) in Pregnancy*, Thieme-Stratton, New York, pp. 4-25 (1981).

23. Grobstein, C., Inductive interaction in the development of the mouse metanephros, J. Exp. Zool. 130:319 (1955).

24. Hsueh, A. J. W., Peck, Jr., E. J., and Clark, J. H., Progesterone antagonism of the oestrogen receptor and oestrogen-induced uterine growth, Nature 254:337 (1975).

25. Iguchi, T., Uchima, F.-D. A., Ostrander, P. L., and Bern, H. A., Growth of normal mouse vaginal epithelial cells in and on collagen gels, Proc. Natl. Acad. Sci. USA 80:3743 (1983).

26. Inaba, T., Wiest, W. G., Strikler, R. C., and Mori, J., Augmentation of the response of mouse uterine epithelial cells to estradiol by uterine stroma, Endocrinology 123:1253 (1988).

27. Kirk, D., King, R. J. B., Heyes, J., Peachey, L., Hirsch, J., and Taylor, R. W. T., Normal human endometrium in cell culture. I. Separation and characterization of epithelial and stromal components *in vitro, In Vitro* 4:651 (1978).

28. Kollar, E. J., Epithelial-mesenchymal interactions in the mammalian integument: tooth development as a model for instructive induction, In: R. H. Sawyer, J. F. Fallon,(eds.), *Epithelial-Mesenchymal Interactions in Development*, Praeger, New York, pp. 27-49 (1983).

29. Korach, K. S., Horigome, Y., Tomooka, Y., Yamashita, S., Newbold, R. R., McLachlan, and J. A., Immunodetection of estrogen receptor in epithelial and mesenchymal tissues of the neonatal mouse uterus, Proc. Natl. Acad. Sci. USA 85:3334 (1988).

30. Kratochwil, K. and Schwartz, P., Tissue interaction in androgen response of embryonic mammary rudiment of mouse: Identification of target tissue of testosterone., Proc. Natl. Acad. Sci. USA 73:4041 (1976).

31. Krueger, W. A., Bo, W. J., and Garrison, B. M., DNA replication in the epithelium of rat vagina and lower cervix following estrogen-progesterone treatment, J. Anat. 139:123 (1974).

32. Leavitt, W. W., Cobb, A. D., and Takeda, A., Progesterone-modulation of estrogen action: rapid down regulation of nuclear acceptor sites for the estrogen receptor, Adv. Exp. Med. Biol. 230:49 (1987).

33. Lejeune, B. and Leroy, F., Role of the uterine epithelium in inducing the decidual cell reaction., Prog. Reprod. Biol. 7:92 (1980).

34. Lejeune, B., VanHoeck, J., and Leroy, F., Transmitter role of the luminal uterine epithelium in the induction of decidualization in rats, J. Reprod. Fertil. 61:235 (1981).

35. Lisczak, T. M., Richardson, G. S., MacLaughlin, D. T., and Kornblith, P. L., Ultrastructure of human endometrial epithelium in monolayer culture with and without steroid hormones, *In Vitro* 13:344 (1977).

36. Markaverich, B. M., Upchurch, S., and Clark, J. H., Progesterone and dexamethasone antagonism of uterine growth: a role for a second nuclear binding site for estradiol in estrogen action, J. Steroid Biochem. 14:125 (1981)

37. Martin L., Estrogens, anti-estrogens and the regulation of cell proliferation in the female reproductive tract *in vivo*, In: J. A. McLachlan,(ed.), *Estrogen in the Environment*, Elsevier/North-Holland, New York, p.103 (1980).

38. Martin, L., Finn, C. A., and Trinder, G., Hypertrophy and hyperplasia in the mouse uterus after oestrogen treatment: an autoradiographic study, J. Endocr. 56:133 (1973).

39. McLachlan, J. A., DiAugustine, R. P., and Newbold R. R., Estrogen induced uterine cell proliferation in organ culture is inhibited by antibodies to epidermal growth factor, Proc 69th Annual Meeting Endocrine Soc., Indianapolis, Endocrinology 120 (suppl):abstr 313 (1987).

40. Moll, R., Franke, W. W., Schiller, D. L., Geiger, B., and Krepler R., The catalog of human cytokeratin polypeptides: patterns of expression of specific cytokeratins in normal epithelia, tumors, and cultured cells, Cell 31:11 (1982).

41. Mori, T., Nagasawa, H., and Nakajima Y., Strain-difference in the induction of adenomyosis by intrauterine pituitary grafting in mice, Lab. Animal Sci. 32:40 (1982).

42. Murphy, L. J., Murphy, L. C., and Friesen H. G., A role for the insulin-like growth factors as estromedins in the rat uterus, Trans. Assoc. Am. Physicians 100:204 (1987).

43. Ogasawara, Y., Okamoto, S., Kitamura, Y., and Matsumoto, K., Proliferative pattern of uterine cells from birth to adulthood in intact neonatally castrated, and/or adrenalectomized mice, assayed by incorporation of (^{125}I)iododeoxyuridine, Endocrinology 113:582 (1983).

44. Okulicz, W. C., Evans, R. W., and Leavitt, W. W., Progesterone regulation of the occupied form of nuclear estrogen receptor, Sci. 213:1503 (1981).

45. Prasad, M. R. N., Sar, M., and Stumpf, W. E., Regional differences between nuclear concentration of [^{3}H]estradiol and [^{3}H]progesterone and their action on the uterus of rat during delayed implantation, J. Exp. Zool. 197:71 (1976).

46. Sariola, H., Ekblom, P., and Henke-Fahle, S., Embryonic neurons as in vitro inducers of differentiation of nephrogenic mesenchyme, Dev. Biol. 132:271 (1989).

47. Sawyer, R. H., The role of epithelial-mesenchymal interactions in regulating gene expression during avian scale morphogenesis, In: R. H. Sawyer, J. F. Fallon,(eds.) Epithelial-Mesenchymal Interactions in Development, Praeger, New York, pp. 115-146 (1983).

48. Saxen, L., Directive versus permissive induction: a working hypothesis. In: J. W. Lash, M. M. Burger, (eds.), Cell and Tissue Interactions, Raven Press, New York, pp. 1-9 (1977).

49. Scully, R. E. and Welch, W. R., Pathology of the human female genital tract after prenatal exposure to diethylstilbestrol, In: A. L. Herbst, H. A. Bern, (eds.), Developmental Effects of Diethylstilbestrol (DES) in Pregnancy, Thieme-Stratton, New York, pp. 26-45 (1981).

50. Smith, B. T., Floros, J., and Post, M.,Hormonal/intercellular control of lung maturation, Prog. Clin. Biol. Res. 226:141 (1986).

51. Stancel, G. M., Gardner, R. M., Kirkland, J. L., Lin, T. H., Lingham, R. B., Loose-Mitchell, D. S., Mukku, V. R., Orengo, C. A., and Verner, G., Interactions between estrogen and EGF in uterine growth and function, Adv. Exp. Med. Biol. 230:99 (1987)

52. Stewart, P. J. and Webster R. A., Intrauterine injection of cholera toxin induces estrogen-like uterine growth, Biol. Reprod. 29:671 (1983).

53. Sugimura, Y., Cunha, G. R., and Bigsby, R. M., Androgenic induction of DNA synthesis in prostatic glands induced in the urothelium of testicular feminized (Tfm/Y) mice, Prostate 9:217 (1986).

54. Sun, T.-T., Tsen, S. C. G., Huang, A. J.-W., Cooper, D., Schermer, A., Lynch, M. H., Weiks, R., and Eichner, R., Monoclonal antibody studies of mammalian epithelial keratins: a review, Ann. NY Acad. Sci. 455:307 (1985).

55. Tachi, C., Tachi, S., and Linder, H. R., Modification by progesterone of oestradiol-induced cell proliferation, RNA synthesis and oestradiol distribution in the rat uterus, J. Reprod. Fert. 31:59 (1972).

56. Taguchi, O., Bigsby, R. M., and Cunha, G. R., Estrogen responsiveness and the estrogen receptor during development of the murine female reproductive tract, Develop. Growth & Differ. 30:301 (1988).

57. Thompson, N. L., Flanders, K. C., Ellingsworth, L. R., Roberts, A. B., and Sporn, M. B., Cell type specific expression of transforming growth factor beta in neonatal and adult mouse tissue, J. Cell. Biochem. suppl. 12A:D125 (1988).

58. Tomooka, Y., DiAugustine, R. P., and McLachlan, J. A., Proliferation of mouse uterine epithelial cells *in vitro*, Endocrinology 118:1011 (1986).
59. Unsworth, B. and Grobstein, C., Induction of kidney tubules in mouse metanephrogenic mesenchyme by various embryonic mesenchymal tissues, Dev. Biol. 21:547 (1970).
60. Webster, R. A., Zaloudek, C. J., Inman, B. C., and Stewart, P. J., Estrogen-like stimulation of uterine ornithine decarboxylase by cholera toxin, Am. J. Physiol. 246:E288 (1984).
61. Yamashita, S. and Korach, K., A modified immunohistochemical procedure for the detection of estrogen receptor in mouse tissues, Histochem. 90:325 (1989).

Questions

Dr. Bern: There is a lot of evidence of EGF in the genital tract. Dr. Iguchi and Dr. Aderig have recently shown in preliminary studies that appreciable concentrations of EGF receptors are found in the uterus and vagina (poster session). The problem is that we don't know where the receptor is since we use whole organ analysis which means in epithelium or fibromuscular wall or the vascular endothelium. Where is it secreted?

Dr. Bigsby: I think Dr. Stancel's presentation will address this matter. However, I'd like to comment on that. The problem with EGF is that, for example, in McLachlan's group it appears that the EGF is being produced by the epithelial cells. Thus, it may not be a good candidate for a stromal to epithelial cell mediator. There are not many candidates for stromal to epithelial cell interactions in any developing system. Only recently have such mediators been isolated. In the August issue of Science, KGF (keratinocyte growth factor) has been identified as a stromal factor produced only by mesenchymal cells and acts only on epithelial cells and so perhaps there are others.

Dr. Glasser: I want to thank you for doing something which is not only indicating the differences in strain but also indicating the difference in developmental age of the animal which is also important, because neonatal uterus to me is a different ball game than the mature. The other thing I'd like to point out is that in the 70s Martin and Smith did an impressive study in which they reported that uterine epithelial daughter cells are devoid of estrogen receptors. These do not develop receptors until 24-30 hours after the second round of DNA synthesis. If, in fact, you do isolate nuclear and cytoplasmic receptors at that time, you find that the concentration of receptors decreases proportionately to the amount of proliferation.

Dr. Leavitt: I have a question about the lack of estrogen receptor staining in the epithelium of the neonatal mouse. In addition to the strain differences is the question of how many receptors do you need in order to get a response? One of the questions I have is that since the progesterone receptor response is an accepted measure of estrogen response, have you looked for progesterone receptors and how soon do they appear?

Dr. Bigsby: We have looked at progesterone receptors and we've shown that there are more progesterone receptors in the epithelial cells than there are in the mesenchymal cells. In the neonatal animal there is an abundance of progesterone receptors, and that goes down with age. I would say that they are there independently of estrogen receptors, which is not a phenomenon unheard of.

Dr. Leavitt: But if you give estrogen to those animals they will respond (with progesterone receptor synthesis)?

Dr. Bigsby: I don't know if the progesterone receptor responds but it's already very high (as shown in the slide).

Dr. Brenner: I would like to comment on the cytochemical work that I've done in the primates, if estrogen receptor is undetectable in the cells then estrogen treatment will not induce progesterone receptor in those cells. When the cell population begins to develop estrogen receptor then estrogen will induce those cells. Whenever we find no detectable estrogen receptor by immunocytochemistry we find no detectable progesterone receptor in those cells of animals induced by estrogen. These are two distinct cases.

Dr. Leavitt: So that is the population of progesterone receptors which are independent of estrogen stimulation in terms of up regulation, and that's why all cell types don't develop progesterone receptors in response to estrogen?

Dr. Brenner: No, what I'm saying is that when I don't detect estrogen receptors by immunocytochemistry those cells do not contain progesterone receptors.

Dr. Bigsby: I think we need to be careful since we are talking about different systems, perhaps we all need to get together later.

4

Qualitative and Quantitative Morphology of Induction in Endometrial Epithelium

Lynn A. Lavia
Department of Biological Sciences
The Wichita State University
Wichita, Kansas 67208

Summary

It is now universally recognized that the action of estrogen on its target organ is to induce the release of cellular signals in populations of target organ cells which effect changes in a neighboring cell's hypertrophy, proliferation and differentiation. To study these responses in detail, the mechanisms of action need to be examined on a local, cellular level. Therefore, we have undertaken in recent years to use computerized image analysis to quantitatively identify subpopulations of estrogen-stimulated cells which are hypertrophic, and determine how regions of spatially separated cells respond temporally to estrogen induction. These results clearly show that there are subpopulations in the uterine epithelium which respond differentially to estrogen stimulation. In addition, results of studies of morphological interactions between the epithelial-stromal cells of the endometrium are reviewed which show the regionality of these interactions. These studies are reviewed here in an attempt to integrate this knowledge with literature from the realm of developmental biology which provide some insight into this field. Both the qualitative and quantitative aspects of this work has potential to be of diagnostic importance in the human to more precisely calculate the timing of the preimplantation endometrium as well as to more accurately predict the success of uterine adenocarcinoma management.

Introduction

Estrogen activation of target organs is through the induction of complex paracrine controls of target cells. Paracrine induction might be defined as the process whereby one subpopulation of cells exerts an influence on the differentiation path of a second, closely apposed, subpopulation of cells. Some critical developmental stages of epithelial cell differentiation have been described. For example, recent results reviewed elsewhere in this volume (4) indicate that in developing rodent fetal endometrial epithelium, the underlying stromal cells are required to maintain the "undetermined" phenotype of columnar uterine epithelium. These epithelial cells lack estrogen receptors and appear to be directed by adjacent stromal cells below the basement membrane in a process traditionally termed instructional induction. These epithelial cells commence the production of estrogen receptors in the perinatal period, coincidentally with the development of an independence from the stromal signals originally required for phenotypic maintenance and thus, pass through a critical juncture called determination (see 4). It might be argued that epithelial cells after that time respond to estrogen in a characteristically "adult" manner. That is, these cells are assumed to respond permissively to estrogen induction - dividing and differentiating independently. Whether this induction is the result of stromal-epithelial interactions is not known because experimental details of these interactions have not been obtained. Morphological evidences of interactions in other systems have been described (see below). The plasticity of the adult uterus suggests that similar processes may also be involved in the proliferation and maturation of the endometrium. This review documents recent work in our lab which shows some of the morphological changes at the stromal-epithelial interface of uterine luminal epithelial cells stimulated by estrogens which correlate with markers of epithelial cell hypertrophy (determined by image analysis). In this review, attention will be focused on these functional changes in subpopulations which occur in determined "residual" uterine luminal epithelial cells remaining after ovariectomy, which are permissively induced by estrogen.

In addition to the work on the rodent, recent work on stromal-epithelial interactions in the human cycling adult endometrium as well as image analysis of nuclear size is reviewed. The results of this work will be integrated into the overall understanding of uterine endometrial epithelial cell differentiation and interactions.

Materials and Methods

Animals and estrogen treatment

Mature Sprague-Dawley rats (SASCO, Omaha, NE) 3-4 months of age (200-300 gm) were ovariectomized 2 weeks before use. Estradiol-17β (E2) was administered using Alza (Palo Alto, CA) osmotic minipumps (model #2001) implanted subcutaneously into the nuchal region of the rat under anesthesia. Pumps have been previously shown (7) to reproducibly elevate estrogen blood levels over an extended period. Pumps were loaded with E2 dissolved in polyethylene glycol. They were then incubated in sterile saline at 38°, 24 hours before implantation to insure consistent pumping rates. Animals were sacrificed at indicated times, uteri removed and weighed, and then used for assays. For microscopy, the distal portion of the horn was used. Four to five animals were used for each time point. Control animals were ovariectomized sham-operated rats sacrificed at the zero hour time point. The luminal surface epithelium was primarily used in these studies since in the rodent, there are relatively few glands (Figures 1-3).

Feulgen staining and video digitization

This was done according to the method of Lavia (23,24-27). The Feulgen stain-Schiff's reagent was made up according to the method outlined in Sheehan and Hrapchak (61). The optimization of the stain (both hydrolysis and stain time) was performed (26) for the uteri of both control (ovariectomized rat sacrificed at time zero) and E2-treated rats since atrophic nuclei such as found in ovariectomized rat luminal epithelium have different characteristics than hypertrophic epithelium. This has been reported for cells in different states of differentiation in other systems (2,51). The video camera (Dage-MTI 65 series, with Newvicon tube-automatic gain control disabled, black level at zero) was attached to the microscope trinocular stem and interfaced to the microcomputer through a 512 x 512 pixel analog/digital converter board (Imaging Technology Inc., Woburn, MA). The software measuring program used was Image Measure (c) by Microscience (Federal Way, WA). The measurement window was localized on a second monitor utilizing an overlay program driven by a mouse on the interfaced digitizer tablet. The system was calibrated and tested for: 1) linearity of light response over the density range measured; 2) repeated measurement coefficient; 3) shading distortion; 4) glare; and, 5) system resolution loss (19,26). Total magnification at the camera lens was 375x, using an oil immersion 100x objective with matched condenser lens. Only a nucleus which contained 90%+ of its area above a fixed density threshold was measured, at its maximum diameter. A minimum of three sections per animal were examined, with at least 100 cells per section counted, chosen at random.

This procedure was similar to that detailed in the staining kit from Abbott Laboratories, unless noted otherwise. Upon removal, the uterus was blotted and immediately placed in

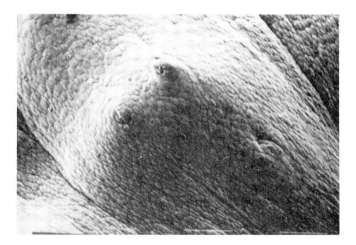

Figure 1. A scanning electron micrograph of the luminal epithelial surface of the mesometrium of a rat uterus after treatment with estrogen. The mouths of glands are seen at the apex of the raised areas. The texture of the surface is due to the presence of turgid epithelial cells (Bar length = 100 μm).

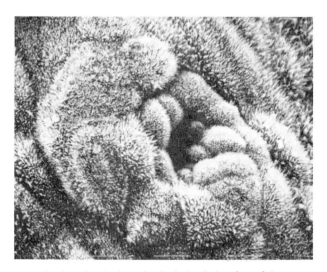

Figure 2. A higher magnification of a gland opening in the luminal surface of the uterus seen in Figure 1 (Bar length = 10 μm).

Tissue preparation for estrogen receptor staining

OCT on a cryostat chuck, then frozen using liquid freon. Tissue was sectioned at 4-6 μm in cryostat. Cryostat sections were thaw-mounted on gelatin-coated glass slides containing central areas for tissue surrounded by a film of teflon/silicone (2 slides/animal). Sections were immediately fixed without drying in 3.7% formaldehyde-PBS (phosphate buffered saline) for 10-15 minutes and transferred to methanol (-10 to -25°) for 5 min. They were then transferred to acetone (-10 to -25°) for 3 min, rinsed in PBS for 4 to 6 min. Excess PBS was removed from the specimen. The slides were flooded with 10% normal goat serum in PBS for 10 minutes to reduce the nonspecific staining of primary antibody. The primary antibody (Abbott, H222) was applied to the tissue at a concentration approaching 20 μg of protein/ml in 10% normal goat serum in PBS. At least one of a series of control primary antibodies was applied to adjacent serial sections from each specimen studied. Slides were washed with PBS two times for 5 minutes each, then blotted. Sections were incubated for 30 minutes with a 1:200 dilution of preabsorbed mouse IgG bridging antibody (Vector Laboratories, Inc, Burlingame, CA) in PBS, with 1:66 dilution of normal goat serum. Slides were washed two times with PBS for 5 minutes each. PAP complex was added dropwise to the sample, left on for 30 min and washed with PBS two times (5 min each). The slides were then flooded with 0.5 meq/ml of 3,3'- diaminobenzidine tetrahydrochloride (DAB-Sigma Chemical Co., St Louis, MO) in 0.05 M Tris Hcl, pH 7.6, 0.01% hydrogen peroxide for 10 minutes at room temperature for visualization. The sections were then washed in deionized distilled water, dehydrated and mounted with Permount and cover slipped with premium quality, #1 thickness cover glass. Preabsorbed mouse anti-rat secondary antibody was used to quench background staining.

Transmission electron microscopy

Tissue processing for transmission electron microscopy was as follows (21). Uterine tissue sections were minced into 1-2 mm pieces and fixed in 3% glutaraldehyde in phosphate buffer (350 mOsm, pH 7.4) for 1 hour. Tissue was rinsed several times in Millonig's buffer. Tissue was post-fixed in 2% osmium tetroxide in phosphate buffer (350 mOsm, pH 7.4) for 1 hour. Tissue was dehydrated through a series of increasing strengths of ethanol. Tissue was then infiltrated in 1:1 propylene oxide:Epon/Araldite for 3 hours at room temperature. Blocks were polymerized in Epon/Araldite at 38° C for 24 h, then at 60 C° for 24 hours. Blocks were sectioned at 50 nm and stained with paragon (63), for light microscopy orientation. Ultrathin sections (50-60 nm) were stained in uranyl acetate for 5 minutes, then in lead citrate for 5 min (53,68). Sections were placed on copper grids and examined.

Statistics

Statistical differences between time points were evaluated using ANOVA followed by Duncan's Multiple Range Test (20). Differences were considered significant when $p < 0.05$.

Results and Discussion

Identification of estrogen-induced hypertrophic cells

Following ovariectomy of the adult cycling animal the endometrium undergoes regression with a subsequent loss of estrogen-dependent endometrial epithelial cells and a corresponding decrease in uterine diameter. Estrogen replacement prompts three major changes in these residual, determined luminal epithelial cells. These are: hypertrophy (characterized on the cellular level by increases in cell size, ribosomal content, etc.), proliferation, and maturation. An extensive literature has catalogued changes in the uterine as well as epithelial layer DNA synthesis, mitotic indices and proliferation rates (9,13,30,32,50,65). However, little work has been performed on the cell population aspects of the hypertrophic response. Therefore,

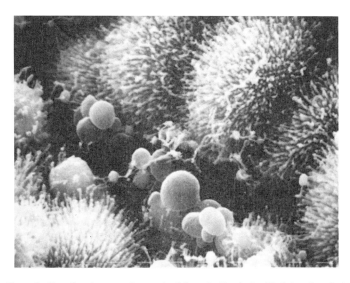

Figure 3. Scanning electron micrograph of the apical luminal epithelial surface during estrogen treatment. Note the secretory particles, released from the epithelial cells (bar = 10μm).

using computer interactive morphometry we undertook to examine cellular hypertrophy in estrogen-stimulated uteri.

In initial studies, we performed morphometric analysis of transmission electron micrographs of rat endometrial luminal epithelial cells, in the ovariectomized and in the estradiol-17β (E2) treated (infusion at the rate of 1.0 μg E2 / 24 h) state (21). Almost all luminal epithelial cells of the ovariectomized endometrium were cuboidal, containing only a few ribosomes found in the cytoplasm. These cells were atrophic. Nuclear areas were measured on electron micrographs using a digitizer tablet interfaced to a computer. Nuclear size was measured in 30-50 cells per animal, 5 animals per group. The mean nuclear area for these atrophic epithelial cells was 28 μm^2, while mean nucleolar area was less than 1.0 μm^2 (56). In contrast to the atrophic cells, many luminal epithelial cells at 18 hours after beginning estrogen infusion were quite columnar, had a substantial increase in numbers of cytoplasmic ribosomes, as well as mitochondria (21). These cells were histologically hypertrophic. Mean nuclear area of the hypertrophic epithelial cells at 18 hours was 36 μm^2, mean nucleolar area was 2.9 μm^2 (both nuclear and nucleolar areas were significantly different than the zero hour control, ovariectomized state). Figure 4 shows the comparison in mean area changes in nuclear and nucleolar sizes for several time points over a 41 hour time period after beginning infusion of E2. These results are similar to and extend those obtained in other studies on the effect of estrogen injections on uterine epithelial cell nuclei (67,69).

In an examination of nuclear area data on individual cells, two additional observations were made. First, we could set a threshold on nuclear area, those cells having nuclear area greater than that size being hypertrophic (as defined above). Second, while mean nuclear size increased throughout the population of stimulated cells, it was evident that not all the luminal epithelial cells were similarly hypertrophic in a single endometrium. However, neighboring cells of those which were hypertrophic, also tended to be hypertrophic, based on nuclear area measurements.

Since mature ovariectomized rat endometrial luminal cells were still in a round of proliferation at 41 hours under this regimen (21), it was not known what effect additional

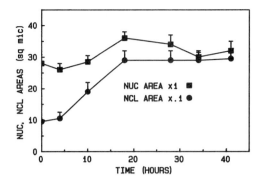

Figure 4. Mean nuclear and nucleolar areas in cells of the endometrial luminal epithelium during infusion of 1.0 μg E2/24 hours. Nuclear size decreased by 4 hours after beginning infusion and increased by 18 hours. Nucleolar size increased by 18 hours. Differences between groups are indicated by separation by a semicolon. Nuclei: 0=10;4;18=28;34=41. Nucleoli: 0=4;10;18=28=34=41 [from Lavia *et al.*, (21), with permission].

time would have on the proportion of cells with hypertrophic nuclei as the hormone-induced full organ differentiation-maturation apparently begins at 3-5 days (17,54). Also, the effect of continuous infusion of different E2 dose rates on nuclear hypertrophy had not been studied, we decided to examine these concomitantly. Therefore, we decided to use different dose rates of E2 over an extended period of time. Due to the tediousness of morphometry using electron micrographs, and the recent availability of PC based densitometry, Feulgen-stained light microscopy specimens were used. This gave similarly accurate measurements in less time and also provided identification of cells in S and G_2 phases of the cell cycle (26).

The image analysis system was calibrated as described in the Materials and Methods, and digitized images of epithelial cell nuclei using various E2 infusion rates and time points were

Table 1. Percentages of hypertrophic uterine luminal epithelial cells at various times under various infusion rates of estradiol-17β. The results are the mean (± S.D.) percentages of hypertrophic cells based on 300 cells counted per animal, 4-5 animals per group. Significantly different groups, based on Duncan's Multiple Range Test (20) are separated by semicolons: 0h; 28h-0.1=28h-1.0=28h-10.0; 96h-0.1; 96h-1.0; 96h-10.0

Time (hour)	Dose Rate (μg E2/24 hour)	Percentage of hypertrophic cells (%)
0	0.0	1 ± 1
28	0.1	14 ± 6
	1.0	15 ± 6
	10.0	15 ± 6
96	0.1	37 ± 9
	1.0	61 ± 12
	10.0	83 ± 3

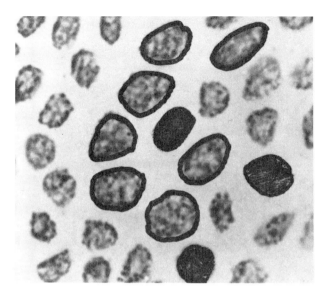

Figure 5. Endometrial luminal epithelial cell sheet. These cells were stained with Feulgen and examined by computer densitometry. Cells with circled nuclei (seven in micrograph) were in DNA synthesis phase (S or G_2) and cells with darkened nuclei (three in micrograph) were hypertrophic, while remaining cells had nuclear areas below threshold.

analyzed. In this study, three infusion regimens were used. These were continuous infusions of 0.1, 1.0 and 10.0 μg E2/24 hours. Animals were sacrificed at 0 (control-ovariectomized group), 28 and 96 hours. The results are shown in Table 1. Regardless of dose, only about 15% of the total number of cells measured (utilizing measurements of 300 cells/rat, 4-5 rats/time point) had hypertrophic nuclei at 28 hours. However, at 96 hours the number of hypertrophic cell nuclei were dose dependent, with a maximum of 84% of the cells being hypertrophic using the 10.0 μg E2 / 24 hour infusion rate.

These results suggested two things. First, that estrogen selectively recruits a subpopulation of the residual, determined, luminal epithelium which hypertrophies relatively soon after treatment, at least by 28 hours. Second, only after cellular proliferation begins does the hypertrophic response become dose-dependent. Again, an examination of the spatial distribution of hypertrophic cells revealed that when one hypertrophic cell nucleus was found, its neighbors tended also to be hypertrophic. This was further evidence that hypertrophic cells were in clusters. In a analogous study Purnell (40) examined mitotic figures in uterine cross sections. He found a statistically greater than random probability that a neighboring cell of a mitotic cell was also mitotic. We have performed a similar study, except instead of using mitotic figures we identified nuclei whose density was greater than 2n (thus being in S or G_2 phase of the cell cycle). Minipumps infusing estrogen were used to stimulate rat uterine luminal epithelial cells for 28 hours (the beginning of DNA synthesis in this model-21). Animals were then sacrificed, uteri were removed and placed in a 1.0% solution of trypsin for an hour. The resulting epithelial cell sheets were spread on slides and fixed, then stained with Feulgen. A typical result is shown in Figure 5. The enlarged nuclei in the micrograph were determined by densitometric analysis of Feulgen-stained specimens to have more than a 2n concentration of DNA, thus, they were either in S or G_2 phase. These cells were arranged in clusters.

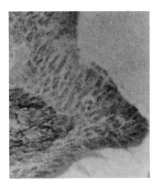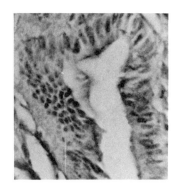

Figure 6. An examination of luminal epithelial cells after treatment with estrogen. These tissues have been stained with H222, an estrogen receptor antibody. The tissue on the left is the control, stained as usual, but without the primary antibody, and counter-stained with hematoxylin for location of nuclei. The tissue on the right has been stained similarly to that on the left, except that the primary antibody (H222) has been added. Note the dark nuclei as well as the heterogenous response in these cells.

These data taken together, suggest that estrogen induces a heterogenous response in luminal epithelial cells of the endometrium and that only a small subpopulation of cells, grouped in clusters, initially hypertrophy. Do these cells have estrogen receptors? For an indirect answer to that, we have reexamined histological uterine specimens from ovariectomized mice. These animals had minipumps implanted (infusing estrogen) and were sacrificed at various times thereafter (Figure 5). Increases in nuclear areas were highly correlated with increases in the density of the Abbott H222 nuclear estrogen receptor antibody staining (24,25). Thus, it was the hypertrophic nuclei which showed an increase in estrogen receptor nuclear stain density. If these receptor results are confirmed in the rat model (which seems likely), that would be strong evidence that this heterogenous response involves cells with an increased number of estrogen receptors seen in the hypertrophic cells of the luminal epithelial layer.

If this is the case, then the question of which stimulates the other will require further work. Thus following estrogen replacement in the ovariectomized rat, the luminal epithelial cells of the ovariectomized endometrium go through a period of synchronization within four hours (nuclear condensation-Fig. 4), then the response became heterogenous. A subpopulation of cells (15%) hypertrophy; these apparently contain increased numbers of nuclear estrogen receptors. It is possible that these "recruited" cells (15%) may be estrogen-stimulated stem cells.

A stem cell (29,36,52) has the ability to divide throughout life, producing stem cells and differentiated daughter cells in an asymmetric division pattern. Stem cells have been tentatively identified in three different types of cell populations: the static cell population, the cell population under stimulated (conditional) renewal, and the permanently renewing population (15).

The stem cell, either because of its spatial position, or phenotype, forms the heart of the basic epithelial proliferative unit (EPU-37,38). Within this unit, in at least some epithelial systems, stem cells produce intermediate cell types, termed transient amplifying cells (TACs), which proliferate rapidly and produce terminally differentiated cells. TACs have been identified in intestinal epithelium (38). It is suggested that at least some of the hypertrophic cells seen after 28 hours (Table 1) may be TACs. There are no universally recognized markers of stem cells, but they do appear to have a slower turnover rate than the rest of the population and have been estimated to comprise 10-20% of the cell population (38), the same approximate number recruited by estrogen to hypertrophy initially. Thus, these hypertrophic cells in the luminal epithelium were tentatively termed stem cells. These

Table 2. Mean nuclear and nucleolar areas of endometrial epithelium in various subphases of the menstrual cycle, in hyperplasia and adenocarcinoma. Each group (subphase) is the mean ± S.D. of nuclear/nucleolar areas from endometrial currettings from 5 women which were assigned to groups on the basis of examination of histology by a pathologist. The groups include: EP = early proliferative; LP = late proliferative; ES = early secretory; MS = middle secretory; LS = late secretory; AH = adenomatous hyperplasia; AAH = atypical adenomatous hyperplasia; G1 = grade 1 adenocarcinoma; G2 = grade 2 adenocarcinoma; G3 = grade 3 adenocarcinoma [portions of data from Roberts et al., (55), with permission]

Endometrial Stage	Nuclear Area (μm^2)	Nucleolar Area (μm^2)
EP	22 ± 4	2.35 ± 0.52
LP	23 ± 3	2.35 ± 0.39
ES	27 ± 4	2.58 ± 0.33
MS	24 ± 3	2.05 ± 0.31
LS	28 ± 5	1.59 ± 0.38
AH	27 ± 6	2.53 ± 0.41
AAH	27 ± 6	2.47 ± 0.26
G1	26 ± 5	2.03 ± 0.24
G2	30 ± 6	2.37 ± 0.65
G3	51 ± 10	3.14 ± 0.50

experiments suggested that the population kinetics in estrogen-stimulated epithelium is indeed complex. Another example of heterogenous response has also been recently described for uterine epithelial cell steroid receptors (71).

This situation is somewhat different in the primate uterus in which recent experiments suggest that cell replacement begins deep within the glands in the cycling primate (35). However, the rodent endometrium is not nearly as glandular as the primate (see Figs. 1 and 2).

Quantitation of epithelial cell hypertrophy in the human endometrium in normal and abnormal states

Quantitation of nuclear area as an index of hypertrophy may also be of value in a more accurate assessment of functional endometrial morphology. This methodology has been applied in this area relatively recently. Earlier ultrastructural studies described the "typical" adult endometrial epithelial cell in different hormone states. These included work on the endometrium of the human (6,12,33,70) in normal cycling, hyperplastic and neoplastic states. Classic studies of the normal cycle have been summarized by Verma (66) who described the idealized endometrial epithelial cell during the menstrual cycle. We have recently completed a quantitative ultrastructural analysis of nuclei and nucleoli in endometrial epithelium during varying subphases of the menstrual cycle as well as during varying stages of hyperplasia and frank adenocarcinoma (Table 2). These results suggest that these types of measurements are of some value, especially for separating early secretory endometrium from other menstrual cycle substages, as well as for separating undifferentiated adenocarcinoma (Grade 3) from other types of adenocarcinoma. However, based on the above results on the rodent endometrium, data from studies of this type need to be reexamined to consider subpopulations of cells, which appear to exist (55,58), especially in light of the fact that induction of cellular hypertrophy and proliferation may be two different functional states (3,8,18,59,64).

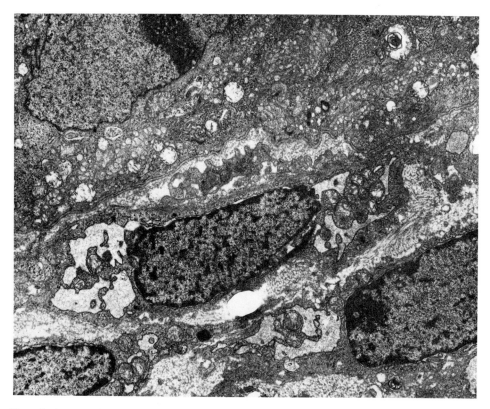

Figure 7. Stromal cell (lower cell) shown below lamina densa (thread-like line below the upper epithelial cells) at 41 hours following minipump implantation (1.0 μg E2/24 hours). Stromal cell is undergoing intense protein synthesis (dilated er).tooth (62) and integument (31) among others. The white area below the stromal cell is an artifact.

Stromal-epithelial interactions during hypertrophy and proliferation

Mesenchymal-(stromal) epithelial interactions are required for organ growth and differentiation in the adult and embryo. Yet the extent of these interactions are not well known, especially in the uterus, although experimental data suggests that there are critical times when interactions occur. In the next sections we will briefly review the experimental literature and describe how more recent morphological data may begin to explain the meanings of these interactions.

Developmental Aspects of Epithelial Differentiation

Morphological studies of the embryological development of the uterus in mammals have been described by Grunewald (14) Norris & Hertig (33), Davies (11) and O'Rahilly (34). While the reader is referred to these texts for details, the main developmental sequence of general mammalian uterine endometrium is recapitulated here as a baseline upon which to examine the complex morphological interactions.

The endometrial stroma and epithelium develop from coelomic mesoderm. Initially, a thickened plate of epithelium develops on the lateral border of the mesonephros. The paramesonephric duct (first identified by Müller in 1825) develops from invaginations in the mesothelial lining of the peritoneal cavity, on the lateral margin of the mesonephros. The

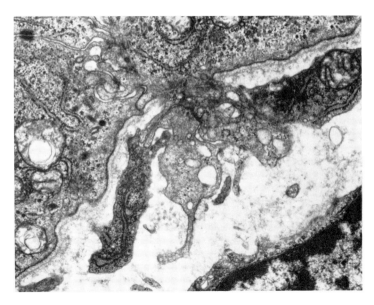

Figure 8. Epithelial cells (left upper) above lamina densa. Epithelial extensions (feet) extend through the lamina densa. Stromal cells are closely apposed on the right and left of the "feet," and another stromal cell body is shown in the lower right portion of the picture [from Roberts *et al.*, (57) with permission].

columnar epithelial cells of this process are presumptive progenitor cells of endometrial epithelium.

The right and left paramesonephric ducts initially grow caudally along the mesonephros and eventually the epithelial cell masses of each duct fuse, followed by fusion of the duct lumen. In this process of organ morphogenesis, epithelial development is apparently controlled by instructive induction of the stromal cells which results in the establishment of a unique phenotype of uterine epithelium. Experimental evidence of the requirement for instructive induction has been described for this period (11,33,34). The signals controlling induction appear to involve extracellular alterations in the basement membrane separating stromal and epithelial cells as well as growth factors released by stromal cells of the uterine stroma, based on comparisons with other systems (16,60).

It is suggested that stromal signals in the above described morphogenetic processes are different than those which appear to control determination. In the rodent uterus, determination occurs later than uterine morphogenesis, as uterine epithelium "learns" that it is columnar uterine epithelium and maintains that phenotype in spite of a transfer to different stroma in recombination experiments. This was originally shown by Cunha and colleagues for the uterus (4). Determination occurs early postnatally in some species of rodents. Besides the functional hallmark of stromal independence, it is suggested that determination is also marked by the appearance of nuclear estrogen receptors in most or all of these epithelial cells. In some systems the control of determination appears to be through the release of either stimulatory or inhibitory stromal signals (16,60). Whether similar signals control this process in the uterus remains to be seen.

The search for these factors is quite important. Recent ultrastructural studies on developing systems also holds clues for the understanding of inductive control mechanisms which may help to differentiate the type of factors required based on spatial distances seen between these cells. An examination of ultrastructural changes at the basement membrane separating stromal and epithelial cells have shown that epithelial and stromal cells have an altered spatial distance between each other during the process of organ morphogenesis. This conclusion is based on studies of embryonic tissues in rodent lung (1,5).

These studies have shown that there are basically three levels of interaction between stromal and epithelial cells, based on spatial distances between these cells. Stromal-epithelial distances greater than 100 nm are termed distant interactions. Those between 20 and 100 nm are termed intermediate interactions. Those less than 20 nm are termed close interactions. Close interactions require a loss of intervening lamina densa (62). In general, these ultrastructural studies suggest that in early morphogenesis there are distant interactions between stromal and epithelial cells, but as morphogenesis ends and epithelial cell terminal differentiation begins, close interactions develop and there is an increase in the number of gap junction complexes between epithelial cells. These results suggest that at least two types of signals are operative during this process. Signals which transverse a relative distance during proliferation and must be chemically stable and those which traverse short distances at differentiation (determination?), which must be more unstable chemically. Similar ultrastructural studies are lacking for the developing uterus. However, morphological studies of the stromal-epithelial interactions have been performed for the estrogen-stimulated adult rat uterus and human cycling endometrium which may be instructive (see below).

Stromal-epithelial interactions in adult endometrium as a result of the permissive induction of estrogen and/or progesterone

Recently, studies of the ultrastructure of stromal-epithelial interactions which occur during permissive induction of the determined "residual" ovariectomized adult rat uterine luminal epithelial cell layer by estradiol-17β have been performed (23). Stromal cells below the lamina densa of the basement membrane still maintained contact with the lamina densa through extended cell processes in the ovariectomized animal; however, in general, stromal cell bodies remained farther than 100 nm from the lamina densa.

Stromal cell bodies migrated to the lamina densa where epithelial and stromal cells became tightly apposed to opposite sides of the lamina densa within 18 hours after implantation of estrogen infusing minipumps (dose rate: 1.0 μg E2/ 24h). By 41 hours after beginning infusion, stromal cells near the intact lamina densa were in the process of marked protein synthesis, as indicated by the dilated endoplasmic reticulum (Figure 7). Thus, stromal-epithelial cell interactions did occur during estrogen stimulation of the adult castrate rat, but all interactions were either distant or intermediate interactions, and the lamina densa remained intact, and in fact, became denser.

In an examination of stromal-epithelial cell interactions of the cycling human endometrium, a slightly different story emerged. In these studies endometrial samples from five women in each of five subphases of the menstrual cycle were analyzed. These included: early and late proliferative, early middle and late secretory subphases (57).

Stromal-epithelial cell interactions were distant during the early and late proliferative subphases, during which time the lamina densa was usually intact. There were occasional gaps in the lamina densa with some epithelial cell processes extending through these openings. Short gap junction complexes were only rarely noted between adjacent epithelial cells during the early proliferative subphase. These increased in size and number during late proliferative phase. In addition, there were complex interactions occurring between epithelial cells and the underlying stromal cells through openings in the lamina densa. Epithelial cell processes occasionally were noted to protrude through the lamina densa. Occasionally, complex cell "feet" were seen which came within 10 nm of stromal cells below (close interaction). Figure 8 is an example of a complex interaction of this type. It has been suggested that there may be some stromal-epithelial cell fusion but conclusive evidence for this is lacking. Multiple epithelial cells appear to be physically involved in this "foot," as gap junctions appear to have formed in the cell foot between neighboring epithelial cells. On occasion, there were intermediate interactions at the lamina densa between an overlying epithelial cell and its underlying stromal cell.

42

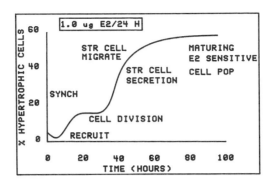

Figure 9. A model of population changes in luminal epithelial cells and stromal cells immediately adjacent. This model shows the effects after implanting a minipump infusing 1.0 μg E2/24 hours. Within four hours after implantation, epithelial nuclei synchronously condense (SYNCH). After this time, approximately 15% of the epithelial cells are "recruited" to hypertrophy as stromal cells migrate to the lamina densa. After the epithelial cells begin to proliferate, stromal cells adjacent to the lamina densa begin to produce protein. Within 96 hours, approximately 64% of the epithelial cells have nuclei which are hypertrophic as the epithelial cell layer begins to mature.point.

The close interactions seen in especially the human endometrium near the conversion of proliferative epithelial cells to glycogenated secretory cells at the time of ovulation suggests that stromal inductive effects are quite important for the terminal differentiation in the epithelial cell layer seen at the time of ovulation in the human. Since at least most of the proliferative cells have estrogen receptors (39), it is assumed that they are determined (see above), and thus, the induction is permissive. However, these studies show that stromal cells continue to exert inductive influences which may affect the ability of epithelial cells to develop normally. In fact, these interactions are not different than those described above for developing systems (see above). It has been further suggested that it is precisely this lack of stromal cell "control" over its endometrial epithelium which may allow hyperplastic and even neoplastic development (12).

The differences between the complex stromal-epithelial cell interactions seen in the human and the indirect, more distant interactions seen in the rat endometrium may be due to differences in the particular system requirements of the epithelium in these species. The interaction differences appear to be related to species differences in function. Therefore, differences in stromal signals should be seen between species. Rat epithelial cells do not become heavily glycogenated and are sloughed at the implantation site (28), whereas, in the human many become glycogenated and do not slough.

An integrated model of the estrogen-stimulated uterine stromal-epithelium cells

A synthesis of the data from the identification of subpopulation of epithelial cells with data on stromal-epithelial interactions is integrated into a working model (Figure 9) of estrogen induction of the ovariectomized endometrium containing residual, determined epithelium. The luminal epithelial cells are largely atrophic at time zero, based on nuclear and cell morphology (although there appear to be some hypertrophic cells present-21). Upon implanting a minipump infusing at the rate of 1.0 μg of E2 per 24 hours, all nuclei condense (trough in % hypertrophic cells at approximately 4 hours). This nuclear condensation suggests stromal signaling has shut down epithelial cell nuclear activity during this time. Then as 15% of the luminal epithelial cells become hypertrophic (stem cell activation?), it is noted that stromal cells have migrated to the lamina densa below the luminal cells. Because of the epithelial-ward migration of the stromal cells, the migration is suggested to be due to the release of epithelial cell factors. That these epithelial cells release factors which control stromal cell activities has been previously postulated (28). As cell division begins (21), more cells become hypertrophic (TACs?), and isolated stromal cells immediately next to the lamina densa begin extensive protein synthesis. Whether this synthesis is of inductive signals or extracellular matrix scaffolding is not known, but even extracellular matrix affects epithelial cell activities (see Damjanov, this volume). By 96 hours, up to 64% of the luminal epithelial cells have hypertrophied. It is not known whether extending the experimental time over a substantially longer period will result in the hypertrophy of essentially all of the luminal epithelial cells, as occurred under maximal dosing (10 μg/24 hours) by 96 hours. It would be quite interesting if an intermediate number of hypertrophic cells were produced by this submaximal dose. These results would potentially have a bearing on research in the area of hyperplastic and neoplastic development in the uterus.

These data raise important issues regarding the number and types of signals which control the activation and differentiation of subpopulations of uterine epithelial cells. Future studies need to more precisely define these morpho-functional relationships and then begin to identify the molecular elements involved. These studies will have an impact on our understanding of both general morphogenesis, estrogen-induced growth, and possibly, control of neoplastic development.

References

1. Adamson, I. Y. R. and King, G. M., Epithelial-mesenchymal interactions in postnatal rat lung growth, Exp. Lung Res., 8:261 (1985).
2. Allison, D. C., Refinements in absorption-cytometric measurements of cellular DNA content, Progr. Clin. Biol. Res. 196:167 (1985).
3. Baserga R., Growth in size and cell DNA replication, Exptl. Cell Res. 151:1 (1981).
4. Bigsby, R. M., Reciprocal tissue interactions in morphogenesis and hormonal responsiveness of the female reproductive tract. In: *Cellular Signals Controlling Uterine Function,* L. A. Lavia (ed.), New York, Plenum Press, (1990).
5. Bluemink, J. G., van Maurik, P., Lawson, K. A., Intimate cell contacts at the epithelial/mesenchymal interface in embryonic mouse lung, J. Ultrastruct. Res. 55:527 (1967).
6. Borell, U., Nilsson, O., and Westman, A., The cyclical changes occurring in the epithelium lining the endometrial glands, ACTA Obstet. Gynecol. Scand., 38:365 (1958).
7. Butcher, R. I., Inskeep, E. K., and Pope, R. S., Plasma concentrations of estradiol produced with two delivery systems in ovariectomized rats, Proceed Soc. Exptl. Biol. Med. 158:475 (1971).
8. Cheng, S. V. Y., MacDonald, B. S., Clark, B. F., and Pollard, J. W., Cell growth and cell proliferation may be dissociated in the mouse uterine luminal epithelium treated with female sex steroids, Exptl. Cell Research 160:459 (1985).
9. Clark, J. and Peck, E. J., Jr., Female sex steroid hormones, Monographs in endocrinology, 40:1 (1979).
10. Cunha, G. R., Bigsby, R. M., Cooke, P. S., and Sugimura, Y., Stromal-epithelial interactions in adult organs, Cell Differ. 17:137 (1985).
11. Davies, J., Comparative embryology. In: *Biology of the Uterus.* Wynn R. (ed.). New York, Appleton-Century-Crofts, p. 13 (1967).
12. Ferenczy, A., Gelfand, M. M., and Tzipris, F., The cytodynamics of endometrial hyperplasia and carcinoma, Ann. Pathol., 5:189 (1983).
13. Galand, P., Leroy, F., and Chretien, J., Effect of oestradiol on cell proliferation and histological changes in the uterus and vagina of mice, J. Endocrinol. 49: 243 (1971).
14. Grunewald, P., The relation of the growing mullerian duct to the wolffian duct and its importance for the genesis of malformations, Anat. Rec. 81:1, (1941).
15. Hall, P. A., Watt, F. M., Stem cells: the generation and maintenance of cellular diversity, Development, 106:619 (1989).

16. Heath, J. K. and Smith, A. G., Regulatory factors of embryonic stem cells, J. Cell Sci. (suppl.) 10:257, (1988).

17. Holt, J. P. and Rhe, E., Rat uterine microbiochemistry: metabolic enzyme activities stimulated by 17-Beta-estradiol are localized in epithelial cells. J. Histochem. Cytochem. 35:657 (1987).

18. Hsu, C-Y. J., Komm, B. S., Lyttle, C. R., and Frankel, F., Cloning of estrogen-regulated messenger ribonucleic acids from the rat uterus, Endocrinology 122:631 (1988).

19. Inoue, S., Video microscopy, New York, Plenum Press, pp. 51-55 (1986).

20. Keppel, G., Design and analysis: A researcher's handbook, Englewood Cliffs, New Jersey, Prentice-Hall, Inc. (1973).

21. Lavia, L. A., Roberts, D. K., Walker, N. J., and Anderson, K., Rat luminal cell nuclear area changes correlated with uterine growth responses induced by a low dose infusion or injection of estradiol-17B. Steroids 45:519 (1985).

22. Lavia, L. A., Miller, B., Anderson, K., and Roberts, D. K., Hormone stimulated changes in nuclear area as determined manually using digitizer tablet compared with video image digitization, Acta Stereologica 6:285 (1987).

23. Lavia, L. A., Walker, N. J., and Roberts, D. K., Morphological examination of endometrial stromal-epithelial interface during estrogen infusion of the mature castrate rat. J. Cell Biol., 105:135a (1987).

24. Lavia, L. A., Miller, B., Anderson, K., and Roberts, D. K., Rat endometrial epithelial nuclear area increases correlate with estrogen dose but nuclear density does not. Cytometry, 9, 25 (1988).

25. Lavia, L. A., Miller, B., Anderson, K., and Roberts, D. K., A comparison of calibrated Feulgen staining on frozen versus fixed, embedded sections: a quantitative assessment of nuclear size, Histochem. Cytochem. 36, 344 (1988).

26. Lavia, L. A., Video microscopy: system calibration for densitometric analysis, BioTechniques, 7:1018 (1989).

27. Lavker, R. M. and Sun, T-T., Epidermal stem cells, Invest. Dermatol. 81:121s (1983).

28. Lejeune, B., Van Hoeck, J., and Leroy, F., Transmitter role of the luminal uterine epithelium in the induction of decidualization in rats, J. Reprod. Fert. 61:235 (1981).

29. Leblond, C. P., Classification of cell populations on the basis of their proliferative behavior, National Cancer Institute Monographs, 14:119 (1964).

30. Lin, T-H., Kirkland, J. L., Mukku, V. R., and Stancel, G. M., Regulation of deoxyribonucleic acid polymerase activity in uterine luminal epithelium after multiple doses of estrogen, Endocrinology 122:1403 (1988).

31. Mauger, A., Demarchex, M., and Sengel, P., Role of extracellular matrix and of dermal-epidermal junction architecture in skin development. In: *Matrices and Cell Differentiation*, Kemp, R. B., Hinchliffe, J. R., (eds.), New York, Alan R. Liss, (1984).

32. Mukku, V. R., Kirkland, J. L., Hardy, M. L., and Stancel, G. M., Hormonal control of uterine growth: temporal relationships between estrogen administration and deoxyribonucleic acid synthesis, Endocrinology 111:480 (1982).

33. Norris, H. and Hertig, A., (eds.), The uterus, Baltimore, Md., Williams and Wilkins (1973).

34. O'Rahilly, R., Prenatal human development. In: *Biology of the Uterus*, Wynn, R., (ed.), New York, Plenum Press, pp. 35-57 (1977).

35. Padykula, H. A., Coles, L. G., McCracken, J. A., King, N. W., Jr., Longcope, C., and Kaiserman-Abramof, I. R., A zonal pattern of cell proliferation and differentiation in the Rhesus endometrium during the estrogen surge, Biol. Reprod. 31:1103 (1984).

36. Papaioannou, V. E., Rossant, J., and Gardner, R. L., Stem cells in early mammalian development. In: *Stem Cells and Tissue Homeostasis*. New York, Cambridge University Press, pp. 49-69 (1978).

37. Potten, C. S., Epithelial proliferative populations. In: *Stem Cells and Tissue Homeostasis*, Lord, B. I., Potten, C. S., and Cole, R. J., (eds.), Cambridge, UK, Cambridge University Press, pp. 317-334 (1978).

38. Potten, C. S. and Morris, R. J., Epithelial stem cells *in vivo*, J. Cell Sci. Suppl., 10:45 (1988).
39. Press, M. F., Nousek-Goebl, N., and King, W. J., Immunohistochemical assessment of estrogen receptor distribution in the human endometrium throughout the menstrual cycle, Lab. Invest. 51:495 (1984).
40. Purnell, D.M., Non-random spatial distribution of mitoses in proliferating rat uterine epithelium, Am. J. Anat. 152:599 (1978).
50. Quarmby, V. E. and Korach, K. S., The influence of 17β-estradiol on patterns of cell division in the uterus, Endocrinology 114:694 (1984).
51. Rasch, E., DNA "standards" and the range of accurate DNA estimates by Feulgen absorption microspectrophotometry, Progr. Clin. Biol. Res. 196:185 (1985).
52. Regaud, C., Etudes sur la structure des tubes seminiferes et sur la spermatogenese chez les mammiferes, Archives d'Anatomie microscopiques et de Morphologie experimentale, 4:101 (1901).
53. Reynolds, E. J., Lead citrate as an electron microscopy stain, J. Cell Biol., 17:258 (1963).
54. Ritter, C., Androgen-stimulated restoration in rat seminal vesicle and prostate epithelial cells, Endocrinology, 84:844 (1969).
55. Roberts, D. K., Lavia, L. A., Freedman, R. S., Horbelt, D. V., and Busby-Walker, N., Nuclear and nucleolar areas: a quantitative assessment of endometrial neoplasia, Obstet. Gynecol., 68:705 (1986).
56. Roberts, D. K., Lavia, L. A., and Walker, N. J., Induction of nucleolar changes in rat luminal cells by injection or low-dose infusion of estradiol-17β, Steroids 51:24 (1988).
57. Roberts, D. K., Walker, N. J., and Lavia, L. A., Ultrastructural evidence of stromal-epithelial interactions in the human endometrial cycle, Am. J. Obstet. Gynecol., 158, 854 (1988).
58. Roberts, D. K., Lavia, L. A., Horbelt, D. V., and Walker, N. J., Changes in nuclear and nucleolar areas of glandular cells throughout the menstrual cycle, Intl. J. Gynecol. Pathol., 8:1 (1989).
59. Ronning, O. W. and Pettersen, E. O., Doubling of cell mass is not necessary in order to achieve cell division in cultured human cells, Exptl. Cell Res. 155:267 (1984).
60. Sharpe, P. M. and Ferguson, M. W. J., Mesenchymal influences on epithelial differentiation in developing systems, J. Cell Sci. (Suppl) 10:195 (1988).
61. Sheehan, D. C. and Hrapchak, B. B., *Theory and Practice of Histotechnology*. Saint Louis, Missouri, C. V. Mosby Co., p. 82 (1983).
62. Slavkin, H. C., Snead, M. L., Zeichner-David, M., Jaskoll, T. F., and Smith, B. T., Concepts of epithelial-mesenchymal interactions during development: tooth and lung organogenesis, J. Cell Biochem. 26:117 (1984).
63. Spurlock, B. O., A new stain for thin sections, Am. J. Clin. Pathol., 46:252 (1966).
64. Stack, G. and Gorski, J., Relationship of estrogen receptors and protein synthesis to the mitogenic effects of estrogens, Endocrinology 117:2024 (1985).
65. Tachi, C., Tachi, S., and Lindner, H. R., Modification by progesterone of oestradiol-induced cell proliferation, RNA synthesis and oestradiol distribution in the rat uterus, J. Reprod. Fert. 31:59 (1972).
66. Verma, V., Ultrastructural changes in human endometrium at different phases of the menstrual cycle and their functional significance, Gynecol. Obstet. Invest., 15:193 (1983).
67. Vic, P., Garcia, M., Humeau, C., and Rochefort, H., Early effect of estrogen on chromatin ultrastructure in endometrial nuclei, Molec. Cell Endocrinol. 19:79 (1980).
68. Watson, M. L., Staining of tissue sections for electron microscopy with heavy metals, J. Biophys. Biochem. Cytol., 4:475 (1958).
69. Williams, T. and Rogers, A. W., Morphometric studies of the response of the luminal epithelium in the rat uterus to exogenous hormones, J. Anat., 130:4 (1980).
70. Wynn, R. A., (ed.), *The Biology of the Uterus,* New York, Plenum Press (1989).
71. Zaino, R. J., Clarke, C. L., Feil, P. D., and Satyaswaroop, P. G., Differential distribution of estrogen and progesterone receptors in rabbit uterus detected by dual immunofluorescence, Endocrinology, 125:2728 (1989).

Questions

Dr. Bigsby: Lynn, one of the first slides you showed was a stromal cell engulfing a degenerating epithelial cell. That brought to mind one of the early responses in the stroma (to estrogen) is the appearance of blood cells, macrophages and eosinophils. When you look at the stromal-epithelial interactions are you identifying fibroblastic type stromal cells?

Dr. Lavia: We have looked at the morphology of stromal cells, and noticed both mesenchymal and blood cells but have not looked at them in any more detail than that. Macrophages are rather interesting, but really hard to identify microscopically, at least using the common staining procedures.

Dr. Bern: I hate to add to the complexity of this, but it seems to me that the picture you present in regards for the need for analysis of stem cells requires one to raise the issue of an analysis of stromal cells, which is also necessary. There must an analogous problem there.

Dr. Lavia: Your point is well taken. Nevertheless, the work here points out the development of a flexible model which allows the examination of regional patterns of epithelial cell response to a signal such as estrogen, and secondary signals such as epidermal growth factor. This is useful in studying cellular and regional growth responses. After all, even neoplasia develops initially as a focal, regional phenomenon.

Dr. Glasser: Implied in the Padykula studies and also in that very interesting study by Lejeune and Leroy is that stem cells for epithelial renewal reside below the basal lamina. Work by Roger Peterson suggests that they can migrate from one compartment to another. The interesting thing about the Leroy study is that when you completely denude (the endometrium of its overlying epithelium) it takes eight days to renew the epithelium. When you do cross sections of the denuded area you can not find anything by cellular morphology or cytokeratin staining which looks or smells like epithelial cells, but there are very suspect cells below the basement lamina. The other interesting thing is that there it requires complete replacement for decidualization. In other words, in seven days, when you have 80% of the stromal lining covered, you cannot induce decidualization. That would seem to me to be a very, very interesting topic. I think, like Helen, that stem cells simply respond to a removal of a signal from the proliferative uterine epithelial cells, mobilize and migrate and populate.

Dr. Lavia: Your point is also well taken. Certainly stromal components are important, as in the cervical reserve cell. But I think the response is different in both situations. The Lejeune study removed the epithelial cells which completely changes the epithelial-stromal relationship which was present developmentally (see above). We studied the intact system, which led to an examination of normal recruitment processes. Also interesting is a set of studies by Trelsted who looked at Muellerian duct regression in the male. He found migration of epithelial cells into the stroma. This is an antithesis of what you have said. Which way are we going in the normal situation? Maybe we're going both ways. However, we have not tried to identify cells migrating through the basal lamina.

5

Interactions of Estrogens, Protooncogenes and Growth Factors

G.M. Stancel[1], C. Chiappetta[1], R.M. Gardner[1], S.M. Hyder[1], J.L. Kirkland[2], T.H. Lin[2], R.B. Lingham[1], D.S. Loose-Mitchell[1], V.R. Mukku[1], and C.A. Orengo[1]
Department of Pharmacology, University of Texas Medical School at Houston[1]
Division of Endocrinology, Department of Pediatrics, Baylor College of Medicine[2]
Houston, Texas   77225

Summary

The uterus contains EGF receptors and these are regulated *in vivo* by estrogens. This regulation occurs at the transcriptional level, at least in part. Treatment of immature rats with estradiol also increases uterine levels of several nuclear protooncogenes including c-*fos* and c-*myc*. Considerable evidence suggests that this regulation occurs via interaction of occupied tissue estrogen receptors with an estrogen responsive element located in the 5' upstream region of the fos gene. Based on these results and the work of other laboratories, we propose an overall model for the estrogen control of uterine growth which is similar to the competence/progression model of growth postulated for cultured fibroblasts. In this model the induction of nuclear protooncogenes, which presumably serve as transcription factors, and peptide growth factors/receptors are two distinct mechanisms for amplifying the signal resulting from the interaction of estrogen with its cognate receptor.

Introduction

It has been known for many years that estrogens play a key role in regulating the growth and function of the uterus and other target tissues. Until the 1960's, however, there was little solid information available about the cellular and molecular mechanisms by which estrogens produced these effects. The pioneering studies of Jensen's and Gorski's groups identified the now classical estrogen receptor present in the uterus and other cells that respond to the hormone (see 24, 19, for reviews). Since these receptors were present in the uterus, it seemed reasonable that the simple interaction of the hormone with these macromolecules might initiate events which were both necessary and sufficient to produce the uterine growth response. This possibility stimulated a great deal of research on the structure and properties of steroid receptors, the interactions of receptors with genomic elements, and the activation of individual genes by these receptors. These studies have led to tremendous advances in our understanding of gene activation by steroids (4, 52), but it has been more difficult to define the precise mechanism of growth regulation by estrogens.

This difficulty in defining the mechanism(s) of growth control was emphasized historically by the inability of many groups to obtain the expected growth of cultured cells in response to estrogens alone. Furthermore, Clark's group made the important observation that estrogen stimulated uterine growth was unlikely to be a simple cascade of events resulting from a single hormone-receptor interaction (2). These, and other observations, led us and others to reconsider the straightforward mechanism(s) noted above by which estrogens regulate uterine growth.

Initially, we thought that another hormone(s) might somehow interact with estradiol to stimulate tissue growth. As a first approach to this problem, we examined the uterine response to the steroid in hypophysectomized animals (2). That study did, in fact, illustrate that uterine growth was diminished in the absence of the pituitary. Further studies showed that the effect was due to removal of TSH and a decrease in circulating thyroid hormone levels (14, 26). These studies illustrated that, in the absence of thyroid hormone, estrogens could stimulate many so-called "early" uterine responses (e.g., wet weight and glucose metabolism) but could not stimulate tissue DNA synthesis and cell division. In attempts to elucidate the cellular basis for this defect, we could not demonstrate any differences in the levels, properties or characteristics of uterine estrogen receptors in hypothyroidism; and, as noted above, some uterine responses occurred normally in the absence of a functional thyroid gland.

Taken together, these observations suggested to us the following hypothesis. Estrogens, acting via an estrogen receptor mechanism, stimulate a quiescent cell to a "state" which is capable of progressing toward DNA synthesis. This progression, however, requires the additional stimulus of a polypeptide growth factor working in concert with estrogens. Our previous observations could then be explained if such a hypothetical growth factor and/or its receptor was regulated jointly by thyroid hormone and estrogen. To test this hypothesis, we decided to take the following experimental approach: (1) determine if the uterus contains receptors for peptide growth factors; (2) determine if such growth factors and/or their receptors are regulated by estrogens and thyroid hormone; (3) determine if levels of such growth factors and/or their receptors are correlated with estrogen-induced growth; and, (4) determine if selective manipulation of such growth factors and/or their receptors could alter estrogen-induced growth.

At this point, we had to decide what growth factors to investigate, and our initial efforts were focused on EGF receptors. The stimulus for investigating EGF was that this peptide was first purified on the basis of bioassays measuring incisor eruption and precocious eyelid opening in the mouse (10). These two developmental responses were also known to be affected by the thyroid status of neonatal animals (21). Whether this logic is correct is, of course, unknown, but the uterus did in fact turn out to contain EGF receptors (34,35).

Our subsequent work demonstrated that these uterine EGF receptors were regulated acutely by estrogen treatment (35) and varied throughout the estrous cycle in parallel with plasma estrogens (17). These receptors are present in the uterine epithelium, stroma and myometrium (30). Other recent studies have shown that this regulation is likely to be at the transcriptional level, at least in part, since estrogens elevate steady-state mRNA levels of the uterine EGF receptor (31).

It seemed logical at this point to next investigate uterine responses that could conceivably be activated via an EGF receptor dependent pathway. At about this time, virologists had made a number of breakthroughs in identifying retroviral oncogenes, and it soon became obvious that: (1) nontransformed cells contained analogs (so called protooncogenes or cellular oncogenes) of viral oncogenes; (2) some of these protooncogenes were either growth factors or growth factor receptors; and (3) some growth factors stimulated protooncogene expression (11, 7). These findings suggested that protooncogenes and growth factors play an important role in the growth and function of normal cells. In particular, several groups demonstrated that EGF stimulated the expression of the protooncogene c-*fos* in a variety of cultured cells (1). C-*fos* is the cellular analog of the v-*fos* oncogene originally identified in a murine osteosarcoma causing virus. This gene codes for a protein of 55 kD molecular weight which is modified post-translationally to a 62 kD form. This protein is localized in the cell nucleus, can bind to DNA, and appears to act as a transcription factor for the regulation of other genes (1).

Our idea was thus that estrogen would elevate the level of uterine EGF receptors. These in turn would be activated by endogenous EGF which is present in the tissue (12), and the resultant cellular signal would activate expression of the c-*fos* gene. Consequently, we administered estrogen to animals, isolated uterine RNA samples, and analyzed them for c-*fos* transcripts by blot analysis. These experiments illustrated that c-*fos* expression was dramatically increased by estrogen treatment, but levels of the transcript increased prior to tissue EGF receptor levels. This indicated that the hormonal regulation of the EGF receptor and c-*fos* genes are independent events.

In this paper we will review our studies on the regulation of uterine EGF receptors and protooncogenes, and present a model of how these individual cellular events may fit into the overall control of tissue growth and function by estrogens.

Materials and Methods

Except where noted, immature female rats (20 days of age) were ovariectomized and allowed to recover for 3-7 days prior to use. Estradiol (40 ug/kg) was routinely administered subcutaneously in 0.5 ml of 95% saline/5% ethanol.

The methods for preparation of uterine membranes, assays for ^{125}I-EGF binding, cross-linking of EGF to its receptor, and the measurement of EGF receptor kinase activity have all been described in detail (34,35).

For measurement of steady-state mRNA levels, animals were anesthetized, uteri were removed and homogenized in guanidinium isothiocyanate. Total RNA was prepared by centrifugation through cesium chloride, phenol:chloroform extraction and precipitation. Agarose gel electrophoresis, RNA transfers and hybridization procedures have been previously described (31, 32).

For measurements of uterine contractility, tissues were removed, the ends of the uterine horns were trimmed, and the remaining tissue suspended in Van Dyke's Hastings Media. Tissues were maintained at 37° and 95% O_2/5% CO_2 was bubbled continuously through the media; total volume of the bathing medium was 10 ml. Spontaneous activity was allowed to subside over a period of roughly one hour, a tension of 500 mg was applied to each tissue, and the recorder was adjusted to establish a baseline. EGF or other agents were then added directly to the bathing medium. Responses reported represent the maximum tension developed during the ensuing incubation. Additional details of these methods may be found in Gardner (15, 16).

Results

Uterine EGF Receptors

Membranes prepared from rat uterus contain saturable, high-affinity binding sites for EGF; typical binding and Scatchard plots are illustrated in Figure 1. The K_d for these binding sites is in the sub-nanomolar range and we have observed only a single class of binding sites in a number of studies. This binding reaction is complete within 30-60 minutes at 0°, and the binding of ^{125}I-EGF is not displaced by insulin, fibroblast growth factor or multiplication stimulating activity. A tyrosine kinase activity is associated with these binding sites and is activated by EGF binding (34, 35).

Localization Of EGF Receptors To Uterine Cell Types

Given the presence of EGF receptors in membranes prepared from the uterus, we sought to determine their cellular distribution. For these studies, uterine horns were removed, slit longitudinally, and incubated immediately in buffer containing labelled EGF $\pm$ excess unlabelled growth factor. After autoradiography, grains are seen clearly over all major uterine cell types: luminal epithelium, glandular epithelium, stroma and myometrium. These grains are largely abolished by excess unlabelled EGF, indicating that they represent specific growth factor binding (30).

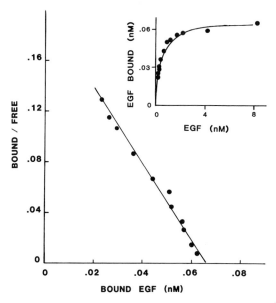

Figure 1. EGF receptors in uterine membranes. The specific binding of ^{125}I-EGF to uterine membranes was measured by a filter binding assay [from Mukku and Stancel (34), with permission].

Regulation Of EGF Receptor By Estrogen

Having determined that EGF receptors were present in uterine tissue, we sought next to examine the regulation of this growth factor receptor by estrogen. For these studies, immature animals were treated with estradiol for varying periods of time before sacrifice and the preparation of uterine membranes. Figure 2 (dashed line) illustrates the results of a typical study, and indicates that EGF binding increases sharply between six and twelve hours after hormone treatment, reaches a maximum at eighteen to twenty-four hours, and then begins to decrease. Other studies indicated that this effect is specific for estrogenic steroids and that the increased binding is due to an increase in the number of EGF receptor sites rather than a change in receptor affinity. Chemical cross-linking experiments using membranes from control and estrogen-treated animals also illustrated that the increase in EGF binding is accounted for by an increase in the 170,000 MW receptor species as visualized by autoradiography after SDS-PAGE (34).

Figure 2 also illustrates the effect of estrogen treatment on steady state levels of the EGF receptor mRNA. It is clearly seen that mRNA levels increase prior to functional receptor levels. We also demonstrated that estrogen could increase EGF receptor mRNA levels in the presence of a protein synthesis inhibitor (31), arguing that the hormonal effect is at least partially transcriptional.

These studies indicated that acute estrogen treatment regulates uterine EGF receptor levels, and we decided to investigate whether physiological levels of ovarian estrogens might also regulate receptor levels. For these studies we simply monitored uterine EGF receptor levels, determined by specific ligand binding, throughout the estrous cycle. As seen in Table 1, there is roughly a two fold change throughout the cycle. The variation shown in Table 1 closely parallels plasma estrogen levels and levels of occupied estrogen receptor throughout the cycle (17).

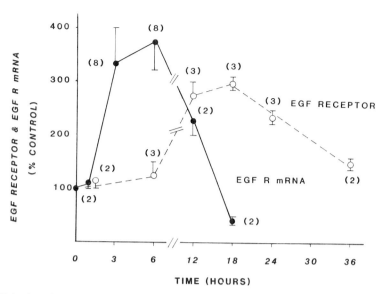

Figure 2. Induction of EGF receptor and its mRNA. Uterine EGF receptor mRNA (solid line) and functional EGF receptor (dashed line) levels after estradiol treatment [from Lingham (31) with permission].

Regulation Of Uterine Contractility By EGF

Our initial interest in EGF and its receptor arose because of the possibility that this peptide might play a role in estrogen stimulated uterine growth. A review of the literature, however, revealed that EGF has other biological activities besides the stimulation of cell growth. For example, EGF inhibits gastric acid secretion (20) and stimulates contractions of vascular smooth muscle (36, 5). This latter report and the observation that the myometrium (as well as other uterine cell types) contains EGF receptors (30, 8), prompted us to investigate the possibility that EGF might affect uterine contractility.

For these studies, segments of uterine tissue from estrogen primed rats were suspended *in vitro* and the contractile response was measured following EGF addition. As seen in Figure 3, addition of EGF caused a prompt response. Within minutes after EGF addition there is an increase in both tone and rhythmicity, and this effect is sustained for several hours (16). Other experiments revealed that this effect: (1) requires estrogen priming *in vivo*; (2) occurs in tissues from mature and immature animals; (3) occurs at EGF concentrations (ED_{50} = 3.5 nM) consistent with a receptor mediated effect; and (4) is abolished by anti-EGF antibodies (16). More recent studies suggest that this effect of EGF is mediated by a mobilization of arachidonic acid and production of uterotonic metabolites by both cyclooxygenase and lipoxygenase catalyzed pathways (16).

This interesting aside illustrates that EGF, and possibly other newly discovered peptide growth factors, may have previously unrecognized effects on the uterus and other tissues.

Regulation of Uterine c-fos Expression

At this point we began to consider possible uterine responses to EGF receptor occupancy, and protooncogene expression seemed a likely candidate (1). Animals were treated with estrogen and total uterine RNA samples were prepared after various times of

Table 1. Uterine EGF receptor Levels Throughout the Rat Estrus Cycle

Stage	EGF Binding[a]
Metestrus	73 ± 10
Diestrus	104 ± 12
Proestrus	151 ± 14
Estrus	73 ± 16

[a]Specific binding of ^{125}I-EGF (dpm bound/μg protein) in isolated uterine membranes. All values were obtained in the early afternoon on the indicated day of the cycle [from Gardner et al., (17) with permission].

treatment. As seen in Table 2, there is a very large rapid increase in c-*fos* expression measured by blot analysis. Much to our surprise this increase clearly preceded the increase in functional EGF receptor levels previously observed (see Figure 2). In fact, the rapidity of this induction clearly suggested that estrogen was directly regulating c-*fos* expression.

A direct effect of estrogen on c-*fos* expression was further suggested by the following observations. (1) Induction is blocked by actinomycin D, but not puromycin (32). (2) Estrogen leads to an increase in c-*fos* expression measured by nuclear run on measurements (51). (3) The 5'-upstream region of the c-*fos* gene contains a palindromic sequence with a high degree of homology to the consensus sequence for the estrogen responsive element, or ERE (32). Our initial reasoning that estrogen up-regulation of the EGF receptor would lead to a subsequent increase in c-*fos* expression was obviously incorrect, but the experiments nevertheless produced the interesting conclusion that uterine expression of the protooncogene was directly regulated by the hormone.

It was also of interest to determine if estrogen would regulate the expression of other uterine protooncogenes. The date in Table 3 illustrates that estrogen also regulates expression of another nuclear protooncogene, c-*myc*. Essentially similar results have already been reported by others (37). In addition to results reported here for c-*fos* and c-*myc*, we have recently observed estrogen regulation of at least two other nuclear protooncogenes, c-*jun* and *jun* B (unpublished observations). These genes are also commonly expressed when cell growth is stimulated by growth factors present in serum (45).

Discussion

Uterine Growth Factors and Receptors

Work in our laboratory has focused primarily on EGF receptors. We have characterized these receptors in uterine membranes (34), determined their cellular localization in the organ (30) and studied their regulation by estrogenic hormones (31, 17). Other workers have demonstrated the presence of EGF in the uterus (18, 12) and uterine luminal fluid (23). DiAugustine (12) has also shown that the tissue contains prepro-EGF mRNA sequences and suggested that EGF levels may be regulated by estrogen. Perhaps more importantly, EGF can affect the growth of uterine cells under a variety of conditions (48, 33, and 6).

It is important to recognize, however, that the uterus contains many other growth factors besides EGF. The uterus contains IGF-1 (38), UDGF or uterine derived growth factor (22), and ULFM or uterine luminal fluid mitogen (46). In addition, PDGF receptors are present in the uterus (43). It is thus possible that a variety of peptide factors somehow interact with steroid hormones to regulate uterine growth and function.

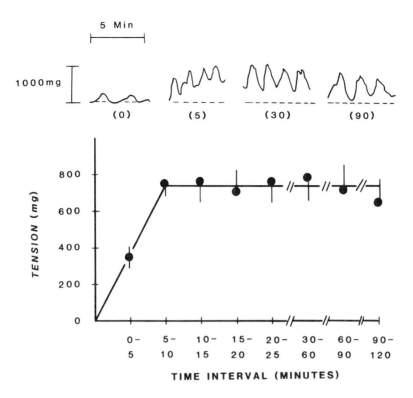

Figure 3. Stimulation of uterine contractions by EGF. (Top) EGF was added *in vitro* to an isolated uterine segment from a mature castrate animal which received estradiol priming *in vivo* for 24 hours prior to sacrifice. The tracings represent contractile activity at the indicated times after EGF addition. (Bottom) Composite showing the maximum tension developed *in vitro* in the indicated time intervals after EGF addition to a series of isolated uterine tissues; N = 6-7 per point [from Gardner (15) with permission].

On the other hand, our studies with EGF induced uterine contractions serve to under-score an important point. Namely, in the absence of definitive proof that growth factors regulate uterine growth in vivo, one cannot rule out the possibility that the real function of these peptides and their cognate receptors is to regulate differentiated function(s) in the tissue. Obviously, these two possibilities are not mutually exclusive.

Protooncogene Expression in the Uterus

We (32) and others (51) have shown that estrogen rapidly stimulates uterine c-*fos* expression *in vivo*. This regulation almost certainly occurs at the transcriptional level, at least in part, for a number of reasons. (1) The increase in expression is very rapid and is blocked by inhibitors of transcription but not translation. (2) The upstream region of the c-*fos* gene contains the palindromic sequence 5'-GGTCT...AGACC-3' at -219/-207 (50), which is very similar to the estrogen responsive element, '5 - GGTCA...TGACC -3', identified in the Xenopus vitellogenin A_2 gene (27). (3) Specificity and dose response studies are consistent with an estrogen receptor mediated effect. (4) Nuclear run-on measurements from Bresciani's group (51) have demonstrated directly an increase in transcription.

Recently, we have obtained more direct evidence that estrogen regulation of c-*fos* expression is a direct effect. We have constructed a fusion gene containing the c-*fos* 5' promotor-regulatory sequences from -351 to +44 linked to a CAT-reporter. (The putative ERE is located at -219 to -207, *vida supra*). We then transfected this construct into GH_3

Table 2. Time Course of c-*fos* mRNA Induction After Estradiol Administration. Ovariectomized rats were treated with estradiol (40 μg/kg) and killed at the indicated times. RNA was prepared and blot analysis performed as described in Materials and Methods. The 2.2 Kb c-*fos* bands of the resultant films were scanned with a laser densitometer. c-*fos* mRNA levels are expressed in relative units based upon control samples present on the same film. Values represent means with the indicated SEM. N represents the number of different samples analyzed at each time point [from Loose-Mitchell, (32) with permission]

Time (h)	c-*fos* mRNA	n
0	1.00 ± 0.22	5
0.5	2.12 ± 0.07	2
1	7.02 ± 1.55	6
3	31.50 ± 8.53	6
6	8.64 ± 1.33	4
12	10.40 ± 0.51	2
15	2.64 ± 0.08	2
18	1.83 ± 0.10	2

cells, a rat pituitary tumor cell line containing estrogen receptors. In this system, nanomolar levels of estradiol rapidly elevate CAT activity, and the magnitude of this increase is the same as that of the estrogen induced expression of endogenous c-*fos* in this cell line (Hyder *et al.*, unpublished observations). While we are in the process of expanding these studies to include deletions of the putative ERE region, these preliminary results establish that the 5' - fos regulatory region contains a "functional" ERE.

While the mechanism of c-*fos* induction by estrogen seems reasonably well established, the role of fos in uterine growth can only be speculative at this time. Recent results on the role of fos in other systems, however, provide some exciting possibilities.

First, fos expression stimulates the transcription of other genes. This is thought to result from the formation of a complex between fos and other transcriptional regulators such as the AP-1/c-*jun* protein, with the complex itself being directly responsible for activation of target gene expression (44, 29, 13, 41, 9). The fos/AP-1 complex could interact with numerous genes having the required AP-1 regulatory sequence. Furthermore, c-*fos* is known to interact with a number of other proteins, the so-called "fos associated proteins" or FAPs (1). This would provide a mechanism for an initial signal from the estrogen receptor:estrogen responsive element (ERE) interaction (at the c-*fos* gene) to be amplified, since the fos/FAP complex could enhance transcription of other genes which do not contain ERE sequences. Such an amplification mechanism would also have a temporal aspect, i.e., the sharp "spike" of fos expression would regulate the times at which these "secondary" genes were expressed in the cell cycle. Such an amplification mechanism would seem well suited to play a role in the massive growth response of the uterus to estrogens.

If fos is acting in the uterus to form such a complex(s) with other nuclear proteins which would then function as a transcriptional regulator, one might expect to also see regulation of such proteins by estrogen. In fact, we have recently observed that estrogen treatment *in vivo* elevates mRNA levels of c-*jun* and *jun* B (unpublished observations), and preliminary studies indicate that this is again a direct action of the steroid.

Second, the c-*fos* gene itself is known to be regulated by a variety of agents other than estrogen, and regulatory sequences other than the ERE are utilized by these other agents to activate c-*fos* transcription. Similarly, the genes activated by complexes such as fos/AP-1 are likely to be subject to regulation by other stimuli, e.g., agents which activate protein kinase C (44, 29, 13, 41, 9). These considerations provide two levels at which estrogen induced responses could be modulated by other stimuli, and vice versa. The first level is the c-*fos* gene itself, and the second level being genes activated by fos-containing complexes. While these suggestions are admittedly speculative they provide a mechanism consistent with our

Table 3. Time Course of c-*myc* mRNA Induction After Estradiol Administration. Ovariectomized rats were treated with estradiol (40 μg/kg) and killed at the indicated times. RNA was prepared and blot analysis performed as described in Materials and Methods. The c-*myc* bands of the resultant films were scanned with a laser densitometer. c-*myc* mRNA levels are expressed in relative units based upon control samples present on the same film. Values represent means with the indicated SEM. N represents the number of different samples analyzed at each time point

Time (h)	c-*myc* mRNA	n
0	1.0 $\pm$ 0.16	43
3	18.9 $\pm$ 0.40	44
6	16.6 $\pm$ 1.13	8
9	8.9 $\pm$ 1.66	8
15	3.2 $\pm$ 1.19	6
27	2.1 $\pm$ 0.11	5
39	0.7 $\pm$ 0.17	3
51	1.1 $\pm$ 0.22	12

current knowledge to allow "cross-talk" between estrogen and other signalling systems.

In addition to fos, the expression of other protooncogenes is activated following estrogenic stimulation of the uterus. These include N-*myc* (38), c-*myc* (38, 49) c-*ras*^{Ha} (49) and erb B (34, 31). Thus, prototypes of all major protooncogene classes (i.e., nuclear protooncogenes, "G"-proteins, and protein kinases) are activated, but the mechanism of these effects is not established as clearly as that of fos induction. Further studies of fos and other oncogenes will hopefully provide additional insights into the physiological, pharmacological and pathological effects of estrogens on normal target tissue.

Overall Uterine Growth in Response to Estrogen

It has been recognized for some time that the regulation of uterine growth by estrogens is a process which is regulated in several stages; and requires more than an initial, transient interaction of the estrogen receptor with an agonist. For example, so called "short-acting" estrogens can interact with the receptor and produce rapid responses similar to those produced by estradiol. These compounds, however, cannot stimulate the complete uterine growth response culminating in DNA synthesis and cell division (2, 3). Endocrinologists have referred to these "stages" of the estrogen induced growth response as "early" and "late effects", "late effects" also being referred to as "true uterine growth". More recently, we have been struck by the general similarity between this model of uterine growth and models of growth in cultured fibroblasts.

In the fibroblast model, the mitogenic stimulation of quiescent cells (in G_0) occurs in at least two major "steps". The first has been termed "competence" and is thought to represent the movement of arrested cells from G_0 into the early portion of G_1, or at least to the G_0/G_1 interface. Movement of cells through G_1 toward S is termed "progression". In the fibroblast system there is a clear demarcation between "competence" and "progression" because the two stages are controlled by different peptide factors. PDGF is the prototype "competence" factor, but alone cannot stimulate mitogenesis. Cells must first be exposed to PDGF and then to a "progression" factor such as EGF or IGF-1 (47, 11, 40). In the uterine system, however, this distinction is not as sharp because estrogen itself seems to be involved in both "early" and "late" effects (2, 3).

The analogy between the two systems is even more striking if one considers that PDGF regulates fos and <u>myc</u> expression in fibroblasts (42) and estradiol regulates fos (57, 32) and <u>myc</u> (49,38) expression in the uterus. While the two stimuli have in common the regulation of these specific genes, mechanistic steps between receptor-agonist interaction and gene expression are clearly different for PDGF and the steroid. Similarly, EGF and IGF-1 are "progression" factors for fibroblasts, and estradiol seems to increase the expression of IGF-

1 (37), the level of EGF (12), and the level of EGF receptors (35, 31) in the uterus. It thus seems reasonable to suggest that the so-called "early" and "late" phases of estrogen action may be analogous in a general way to "competence" and "progression" in fibroblasts.

If one considers fos expression as a marker of the competence state, estrogenic steroids may function via their receptors to elicit competence responses directly at the genomic level. Given our data and the work of others, this seems the most reasonable possibility. While it seems less likely to us, estrogens could conceivably act via a non-genomic mechanism (e.g., conversion of an inactive EGF precursor to an active peptide) which functions through a membrane receptor to stimulate c-*fos* expression. PDGF-like regulation, on the other hand, involves a cytoplasmic second messenger(s) to transmit a signal emanating from the plasma membrane. The basic idea is that steroids and polypeptide growth factors control "competence" by different regulatory mechanisms which converge at a common endpoint(s) such as expression of c-*fos*.

Possible mechanistic analogies between "progression-like" events in the two systems are more difficult to envision. An obvious possibility is that the estrogen-receptor complex directly controls the local production of factors like EGF/IGF-1, and/or their receptors, and these act via autocrine or paracrine mechanisms to control transit through G_1. Unfortunately, it is difficult to evaluate this possibility given existing data on the mechanism of regulation of EGF and IGF-1 by estrogens. Additional studies will obviously be required to evaluate this possibility, and to understand the *in vivo* role of protooncogenes and growth factors in estrogen controlled uterine growth.

Acknowledgments

The authors wish to express their appreciation to Ms. Nancy Womack for preparation of this manuscript. Work from our laboratories was supported by NIH grants HD-08615 (G.M.S.), DK-38965 (D.S.L.-M.), and RR-01685 (Bionet) for computer use, and a grant from the John P. McGovern Foundation (J.L.K.).

References

1. Alt, F.W., Harlow, E., and Ziff, E.B., *Nuclear Oncogenes*, Cold Spring Harbor Laboratory, Cold Spring Harbor, New York. (1987).
2. Anderson, J.N., Clark, J.H., and Peck, E.J., Jr., The relationship between nuclear receptor estrogen binding and uterotrophic responses, Biochem. Biophys. Res. Commun., 48:1460 (1972).
3. Anderson, J.N., Peck, E.J., Jr. and Clark, J.H., Nuclear receptor estrogen complex: relationship between concentration and early uterotrophic responses. Endocr. 92:1488 (1973).
4. Beato, M., Gene regulation by steroid hormones, Cell 56:335 (1989).
5. Berk, B.C., Brock, T.A., Webb, R.C., Taubman, M.B., Atkinson, W.J., Gimbrone, M.A., Jr., and Alexander, R.W., Epidermal growth factor, a vascular smooth muscle mitogen, induces rat aortic contraction, J. Clin. Invest. 75:1083 (1985).
6. Bhargava, G., Rifas, L., and Makman, M.H., Presence of epidermal growth factor receptors and influence of epidermal growth factor on proliferation and aging in cultured smooth muscle cells, J. Cell. Physiol. 100:365 (1979).
7. Bishop, J.M., Viral Oncogenes, Cell 42:23 (1985).
8. Chegini, N., Rao, C.V., Wakin, N., and Sanfilippo, J., Binding of ^{125}I-epidermal growth factor in human uterus, Cell Tissue Res. 246:543 (1986).
9. Chiu, R., Boyle, W.J., Meek, J., Smeol, T., Hunter, T., and Karin, M., The c-*fos* protein interacts with C-*Jun*/AP-1 to stimulate transcription of AP-1 responsive genes, cell 54:541 (1988).

10. Cohen, S.G., Isolation of a mouse submaxillary protein accelerating incision eruption and eyelid opening in the newborn animal, J. Biol. Chem. 237:1555 (1962).

11. Deuel, T.F., Polypeptide growth factors: roles in normal and abnormal cell growth, Ann. Rev. Cell Biol. 3:443 (1987).

12. DiAugustine, R.P., Petrusz, P., Bell, G.I., Brown, C.F., Korach, K.S., McLachlan, J.A., and Teng, C.T., Influence of estrogen on mouse uterine epidermal growth factor precursor protein and messenger ribonucleic acid, Endocr. 122:2355 (1988).

13. Distel, R.J., Ro, H.S., Rosen, B.S., Groves, D.L., and Spiegelman, B.M., Nucleoprotein complexes that regulate gene expression in adipocyte differentiation: direct participation of c-fos, Cell 49:835 (1987).

14. Gardner, R.M., Kirkland, J.L., Ireland, J.S., and Stancel, G.M., Regulation of the uterine response to estrogen by thyroid hormone, Endocr. 103:1164 (1978).

15. Gardner, R.M., Lingham, R.B., and Stancel, G.M., Epidermal growth factor stimulates contractions of the isolated uterus, FASEB J. 1:224 (1987).

16. Gardner, R.M., Goldsmith, J.R., and Stancel, G.M., Pharmacological characterization of epidermal growth factor (EGF) induced uterine contractions, FASEB J. 2:A1143 (1988).

17. Gardner, R.M., Verner, G., Kirkland, J.L., and Stancel, G.M., Regulation of EGF receptors by estrogen in the mature rat and during the estrous cycle, J. Ster. Biochem 32:339 (1989).

18. Gonzalez, F., Lakshmanan, J., Hoath, S., and Fisher, D.A., Effect of oestradiol-17 on uterine epidermal growth factor concentration in immature mice, Acta Endocr. (Copenhagen) 105:425 (1984).

19. Gorski, J. and Gannon, F., Current models of steroid hormone action, a critique, Ann. Rev. Physiol. 38:425 (1976).

20. Gregory, H., *In vivo* aspects of urogastrone-epidermal growth factor, J. Cell Sci.(Suppl.) 3:11 (1985).

21. Hamburgh, M., Mendoza, C.A., Burkart, J.G., and Weil, F., Thyroid dependent processes in the developing nervous system, In: *Hormones and Development*, M. Hamburgh and E.J.W. Banning (eds.), pp. 403-415, Meredith Corp. N.Y. (1971).

22. Ikeda, T., and Sirbasku, P.A., Purification and properties of a mammary uterine pituitary tumor cell growth factor from pregnant sheep uterus, J. Biol. Chem. 259:4049 (1984).

23. Imai, Y., Epidermal growth factor in rat uterine luminal fluid, Endocr. 110 (Suppl): 162: (abstr.), (1982).

24. Jensen, E.V. and DeSombre E.R., Mechanism of action of female sex hormones, Ann. Rev. Biochem. 41:203 (1972).

25. Kirkland, J.L., Gardner, R.M., Ireland, J.S., and Stancel, G.M., The effect of hypophysectomy on the uterine response to estradiol, Endocr. 101:403 (1977).

26. Kirkland, J.L., Gardner, R.M., Mukku, V.R., Aktar, M. and Stancel, G.M., Hormonal control of uterine growth: the effect of hypothyroidism on estrogen stimulated cell division, Endocr. 108:2346 (1981).

27. Klein-Hitpass, L., Schorp, M., Wagner, U., and Ryfell, G.U., An estrogen responsive element derived from the 5' flanking region of xenopus vitellogenin A2 gene functions in transfected human cells, Cell 46:1053 (1986).

28. Knauer, D.J., Wiley, H.S., and Cunningham, D.B., Relationship between epidermal growth factor receptor occupancy and mitogenic response. Quantitative Analysis Using a Steady State Model System, J. Biol. Chem. 259:5623 (1984).

29. Lech, K., Anderson, K., and Brent, R., DNA-bound fos proteins activate transcription in yeast, Cell 52:179 (1988).

30. Lin, T.S., Kirkland, J.L., Mukku, V.R., and Stancel, G.M., Autoradiographic localization of epidermal growth factor binding in individual uterine cell types, Biol Reprod. 38:403 (1988).

31. Lingham, R.B., Stancel, G.M., and Loose-Mitchell, D.M., Regulation of epidermal growth factor receptor messenger RNA by estrogen, Mol. Endocr. 2:230 (1988).

32. Loose-Mitchell, D.S., Chiappetta, C., and Stancel, G.M., Estrogen Regulation c-*fos* Messenger Ribonucleic Acid, Mol. Endocr. 2:946 (1988).

33. McLachlan, J.A., DiAugustine, R.P., and Newbold, R.R., Estrogen induced uterine cell proliferation in organ culture is inhibited by antibodies to epidermal growth factor, Prog. of the 69th Ann. Mtg. of the Endocr. Soc., Indianapolis, IN, p. 99 (Abstr. #313) (1987).

34. Mukku, V.R., and Stancel, G.M., Regulation of uterine epidermal growth factor receptors by estrogen, J. Biol. Chem. 260:9820 (1985).

35. Mukku, V.R., and Stancel, G.M., Receptors for epidermal growth factor in the rat uterus, Endocr. 117:149 (1985 b).

36. Muramatsu, I., Hollenberg, M.D., and Lederis, K., Vascular actions of epidermal growth factor-urogastrone: possible relationship to prostaglandin production, Can. J. Physiol. Pharmacol. 36:994 (1985).

37. Murphy, L.J., Murphy, L.C., and Friesen, H.G., Estrogen induces insulin-like growth factor-1 expression in the rat uterus, Mol. Endocr. 1:445 (1987 a).

38. Murphy, L.J., Murphy, L.C., and Friesen, H.G., Estrogen induction of n-*myc* and c-*myc* protooncogene expression in the rat uterus, Endocr. 120:1882 (1987 b).

39. Murphy, L.J., and Friesen, H.G., Differential effects of estrogen and growth hormone on uterine and hepatic insulin-like growth factor I gene expression in the ovariectomized hypophysectomized rat, Endocr. 122:325 (1988).

40. O'Keefe, E.J., and Pledger, W.J., A model of cell cycle control of sequential events regulated by growth factors, Mol. Cell. Endocr. 31:167 (1983).

41. Rauscher, F.J. III, Sambucetti, L.C., Curran, T., Distel, R.J., and Speigleman, B.M., A common DNA binding site for fos protein and transcription factor AP-1, cell 52:471480 (1988).

42. Rollins, B.J. and Stiles, C.D., Regulation of c-*myc* and c-*fos* proto-oncogene expression by animal cell growth factors, *In Vitro*, Cell. & Dev. Biol. 24:81 (1988).

43. Ronnstrand, L., Beckmann, M.P., Faulders, B., Ostman, A., Ek, B., and Heldin, C.H., Purification of the receptor for PDGF from porcine uterus, J. Biol. Chem. 262:2929 (1987).

44. Ruther, U., Garber, C., Komitowski, D., Muller, R., and Wagner, E.G., Deregulated c-*fos* expression interferes with normal bone development in transgenic mice, nature 325:412 (1987).

45. Ryder, K., Lan, L.F., and Nathans, D., A gene activated by growth factors is related to the oncogene v-*jun*, Proc. Natl. Acad. Sci. USA 85:1487 (1988).

46. Simmen, R.C.M., Ko, Y., Liu, X.H., Wilde, M.H., Pope, W.F., and Simmen, F.A., A Uterine cell mitogen distinct from epidermal growth factor in porcine uterine luminal fluids: characterization and partial purification, Biol. Reprod. 38:551 (1988).

47. Stiles, C.D., Capone, G.T., Scher, C.D., Antoniades, H.N., Van Wyk, J.J., and Pledger, W.J., Dual control of cell growth by somatomedins and platelet-derived growth factor, Proc. Natl. Acad. Sci. 76:1279 (1979).

48. Tomooka, Y., DiAugustine, R.P., and McLachlan, J.A., Proliferation of mouse uterine epithelial cells *in vitro*, Endocr. 118:1011 (1986).

49. Travers, M.T., and Knowler, J.T., Oestrogen-induced expression of oncogenes in the immature rat uterus, FEBS Lett. 211:27 (1987).

50. Treisman, R., Transient accumulation of c-*fos* RNA following serum stimulation requires a conserved 5' element and c-*fos* 3' sequences, Cell 42:889 (1985).

51. Weisz, A., and Bresciani, F., Estrogen induces expression of c-*fos* and c-*myc* protooncogenes in rat uterus, Mol. Endocr. 2:816 (1988).

52. Yamamoto, K.R., Steroid receptor regulated transcription of specific genes and gene networks, Ann. Rev. Genetics 19:209 (1985).

Questions

Dr. Glasser: have you done any *in situ* work, does c-*fos* move around?

Dr. Stancel: In the model system we are using, the immature animal, we have started to do that. We have some results now. It is clear that *fos* is turned on in all the cell types and that is not surprising in this model since all those cell types will divide. We haven't looked at mature, cycling animals, where not all the cells are induced to divide. The epithelial cells make more, the stroma cells make quite a bit, the myometrial cells make some.

Dr. Glasser: What I'm really interested in is a single cell type. Does it compartmentalize within a cell at a particular posthormonal time?

Dr. Stancel: Let me answer this way. We haven't looked at the data to examine it in this way. Let me try to conjure up how the cells looked under the microscope. As I recall in the glandular and luminal epithelial layer where it's easy to see cells, every cell has grains. Now what I can't swear Stan, is whether there are differences in grain densities over individual cells.

Dr. Glasser: Have you tried to castrate these neonates to see if levels decrease and can be restimulated?

Dr. Stancel: That's a really interesting question. The answer is yes. What Stan is referring to is the slides at the end. Those animals received no treatment whatsoever, except DES on day one of life, and we'd let them grow up for thirty days. We then castrate the animals, then wait for a week or so until endogenous levels fall. Then you retreat the animals with DES. What happens? The answer is that animals that got DES treatment neonatally had a large increase in *fos*, and the animals that did not get DES showed the same increases.

6

Expression of Metallothionein Genes in Preimplantation Embryos, Decidua and Placentae

G.K. Andrews[1], S.K. De[1], M.T. McMaster[1] and S.K. Dey[2]
Department of Biochemistry and Molecular Biology[1] and Obstetrics and Gynecology and Physiology[2]
University of Kansas Medical School, 39th and Rainbow Blvd.
Kansas City, Kansas 66103

Summary

Metallothioneins (MT) are cysteine rich, heavy metal binding proteins whose expression can be regulated by a variety of factors, such as metal ions, glucocorticoids, and cytokines. Although little is known about expression of MT genes during early mammalian development, substantial variations in expression of these genes in the fetal and neonatal period occur which has lead to the concept that MT may play important roles during development, such as maintenance of zinc and copper homeostasis and protection from heavy metal toxicity. However, the precise functions of MT are unknown. We have examined expression and regulation of metallothionein genes from the time of fertilization to midgestation. Utilizing the preimplantation rabbit embryo as a model it was determined that MT is constitutively expressed at low levels in the blastocyst (D6), and zinc can induce MT as early as day-4 of gestation just after the morula to blastocyst transition. The mouse embryo also develops the capacity to respond to metal ions by the late morula stage. Therefore, the preimplantation mammalian embryo can alter expression of the genome in response to changes in the levels of metal ions in the oviductal and uterine milieu just prior to implantation. In mice, MT mRNA is present at low levels in the uterine luminal epithelium just before implantation (D4), but upon implantation, MT gene expression is specifically and dramatically elevated in the deciduum (D5-10). In the midgestation placenta, constitutively high levels of MT mRNA are present in the outer placental spongiotrophoblasts. At this stage of gestation, the visceral yolk sac endoderm also actively expresses the MT genes. These results provide the basis for the concept that from the time of implantation to late in gestation, the mouse embryo is surrounded by cells, interposed between the maternal and embryonic environments, which actively express the MT genes. This suggests that MT, and perhaps other stress related proteins, play an important role in the establishment and maintenance of normal pregnancy. Studies of the regulation of MT genes in decidua suggest that embryo derived factors are not involved, but rather that these genes may be regulated in an autocrine/paracrine manner, perhaps in response to the pro-inflammatory process of implantation and decidualization.

Introduction

Metallothioneins (MTs) are cysteine rich, heavy metal binding proteins present in all higher eukaryotes. Two isoforms of MT (MT-I and MT-II) exist which, in the mouse, differ slightly in amino acid sequence and net charge (41). Expression of mammalian MT genes can be regulated by a variety of factors, including but not limited to, essential and toxic metal ions, glucocorticoids, and cytokines (for reviews see: 21,27,28,38).

Cellular Signals Controlling Uterine Function
Edited by L.A. Lavia, Plenum Press, New York

The functions of MT are not all understood (see 28). However, the ability to bind to and be induced by metals suggests that MT plays roles in homeostasis of essential metals (zinc, copper) and in protection from toxic metals such as cadmium. MT has recently been shown to scavenge free hydroxyl radicals (45). The MT genes are also induced in response to inflammation as a component of the acute phase response. Thus, this family of proteins may be involved in the animal's response to a variety of stresses.

The detailed knowledge of the molecular biology of the mouse MT genes, their ability to be transcriptionally induced by such a wide array of signals, and their likely importance in fundamental cellular processes make these genes useful candidates for analysis in the developing embryo and gestational uterus.

Although little is known about expression of MT genes during early mammalian development, substantial variations in expression of these genes in the fetal and neonatal period suggest the importance of MT during embryonic development (reviewed in 48). Specifically, MT-I and II are known to be expressed at high levels in the visceral yolk sac endoderm, and later in fetal and neonatal liver (2,48).

A potential involvement of MT in the development of the preimplantation embryo is suggested by the observations that preimplantation embryonic development can be radically disturbed by exposure to metal ions such as cadmium (50), or conversely, by deficiencies in metal ions such as zinc (25). The potential involvement of MT in the development of the postimplantation embryo is suggested by several observations. In the mouse, placental transfer of cadmium, a potent teratogenic agent, is limited by some unknown mechanism (0.02% of the total maternal dose) (reviewed in 17). Therefore, the placenta is thought to provide a barrier function which protects the developing embryo from this toxic metal (8,17). Normal development of the postimplantation embryo is also influenced by the availability of essential metals, such as zinc and copper in the maternal diet. A deficiency of zinc is teratogenic and leads to abnormal growth and morphogenesis (40,48). zinc has a wide array of physiological functions, many of which can be attributed to changes in the activity of zinc metalloenzymes (13). With these observations in mind, an analysis of expression and regulation of the MT genes in the rabbit blastocyst and the pre- and postimplantation mouse embryo, as well as in the mouse uterus, deciduum and placenta during pregnancy was undertaken.

Materials and Methods

Animals

Adult (7-8 kg, 4-4 1/2 month old) virgin female New Zealand white rabbits were induced to superovulate by injecting, subcutaneously, porcine FSH twice daily for 3 consecutive days. On the morning of the 4th day, rabbits were mated in succession with two fertile bucks and then injected intravenously with 25 I.U. HCG (33). Day-4 and day-6 embryos (Day 1 = 24 h post-coitum) were collected by flushing the uteri and embryos were washed and incubated in the same media under a gas phase of 5% CO_2, 5% O_2 and 90% N_2 at 37° (37).

In order to determine the effects of metal ions on rabbit blastocyst gene expression, day-6 blastocysts were incubated in RPMI-1640 containing 0.3% BSA and 2 mM L-glutamine for 4 h in the presence or absence of various concentrations of $ZnCl_2$ or $CdCl_2$. If day-6 blastocysts were to be pulse-labeled with ^{35}S-cysteine (see below), the BSA was omitted from the final incubation media.

Female CD-1 mice (48 days old; Charles River Laboratories) were mated, and the gestational age of the embryo calculated from the day on which a vaginal plug was detected (designated D1 of gestation). Samples for RNA extraction were obtained as follows: decidua (D8) and decidua/placentae (D10) were dissected free from the uterus, and the embryo and extraembryonic membranes were removed; the visceral yolk sac (D9 to D14) was recovered free of amnion and parietal yolk sac; placentae (D12 to D16) were dissected free from the uterus and extraembryonic membranes. For each experiment tissues from at least three animals were pooled. Pseudopregnancy was induced by mating with vasectomized males, and the decidual reaction (deciduomata) was induced on D4 by injection of 100 μl of sesame oil into the utero - tubular junction. Deciduomata tissue was harvested on D8. Samples were quick frozen and stored at -80° C. Samples for *in situ* hybridization were processed as described below.

Hybridization Probes

A mouse MT-I cDNA, mouse heat shock protein 70 (HSP-70) gene, and a rat placental lactogen-II cDNA (see 4, 15) were inserted into SP6 vectors and used as templates for the synthesis of ^{32}P or ^{35}S-labeled cRNA probes as described by Melton (32). A MT sense strand probe was also synthesized. Probes had specific activities of about 2 x 10^9 dpm/μg. Oligodeoxyribonucleotides (27 nucleotides) complementary to 3' untranslated regions of mouse MT-I or MT-II were synthesized with the following sequences:
MT-I; 5'-GGGTGGAACTGTATAGGAAGACGCTGG-3';
MT-II, 5'-GGTCTATTTACACAGATGTGGGGACCC-3' (41).
These probes were ^{32}P 5' end-labeled using T4 polynucleotide kinase according to the manufacturer's suggestions. These probes had a specific activity of about 2 x 10^8 dpm/μg.

Isolation and Analysis of Total RNA

RNA was extracted by a modification of sodium dodecyl sulfate (SDS)-phenol-chloroform procedures as described in detail previously (4,15). Solution hybridization was used to quantitate MT-I and MT-II mRNA levels according to the methods of Durnam and Palmiter (19) as modified by Omiecinski (36). Details of the procedure have been previously published (15). Total RNA was hybridized with 2 ng/ml of ^{32}P-labeled oligodeoxyribonucleotide (20,000 cpm), and the amount of S1 resistant radioactivity was determined. RNA from control liver and zinc-treated liver served as comparative standards for basal and high levels of MT mRNA, respectively.

Northern blot hybridization was used to analyze changes in the abundance of MT-I mRNA. RNA was denatured and separated by electrophoresis in a 1.5% agarose gel containing 3-(4-morpholino) propane sulfonic acid (MOPS) buffer (20 mM MOPS, 5 mM sodium acetate, 1 mM EDTA, pH 7.0) and 2.2 M formaldehyde as detailed previously (4,15). Following electrophoresis, gels were transferred to nitrocellulose and the blots were pre-hybridized, hybridized and washed as described by Andrews (2). Autoradiographs of the filters were obtained by exposing X-ray film in conjunction with a high-plus intensifying screen.

In Situ *Hybridization*

The methods for *in situ* hybridization have been adapted from procedures published by Angerer and colleagues (5,6,14,16) and are detailed elsewhere (15). Tissues were fixed by perfusion with 4% paraformaldehyde and embedded in paraffin. Paraffin blocks were serially sectioned at 7 μm, and sections were mounted on poly-L-lysine coated slides. Within a given experiment, sections from all experimental samples were mounted onto the same microscope slide, and several slides were prepared. Sections were deparaffinized, rehydrated, and then acetylated (23). Slides were hybridized with ^{35}S-labelled cRNA probes as described (18), and after hybridization, slides were treated with RNase A, washed and autoradiography was performed using Kodak NTB-2 liquid emulsion. Slides were stained lightly in hematoxylin.

Determination of Relative Rates of MT Synthesis

Day-6 and Day-4 rabbit morula and blastocysts (20 to 80 per point) were cultured for 4 h in RPMI-1640 (5 ml) in the presence or absence of metal ions ($CdCl_2$ or $ZnCl_2$). The blastocysts were washed twice in balanced salt solution. Rabbit embryos, and mouse decidua and placentae, obtained as described above, were transferred into cysteine-free Minimal Essential Medium containing 150 μCi/ml ^{35}S-cysteine (specific activity of 1,000 Ci/mM; New

England Nuclear, Boston, MA) and incubated at 37° C for 1 to 3 h. After labeling, the samples were washed twice in PBS and homogenized in an appropriate volume of buffer (22) containing 1% Nonidet P40, 50 mM Tris (pH 7.4), 100 mM NaCl, 5 mM dithiothreitol (DTT) as described previously (4,15). The soluble proteins were recovered by centrifugation and carboxymethylated with iodoacetic acid. Rabbit Day-4 embryos and mouse decidual and placental samples were then incubated at 80° C for 8 min and the heat stable proteins recovered in the supernatant following centrifugation. If required, the heat stable proteins were precipitated with 5 vol of cold ethanol for 18 h at $-20 \cdot$C. Equal amounts of trichloroacetic acid-precipitable radioactivity (as indicated in the figure legends) were separated by 20% polyacrylamide gel electrophoresis in the absence of SDS. Blastocyst samples were not heat treated and were separated by 30% acrylamide - 0.1% SDS gel electrophoresis. Gels were fixed and stained with coomassie blue and radioactive proteins detected by fluorography. Purified carboxymethylated MT served as a reference standard.

Results

Expression of MT Genes in the Preimplantation Embryo

We initially chose to study MT gene expression in the preimplantation rabbit blastocyst (day-4 & day-6 of gestation), because rabbit embryos at these stages have many more cells than do the preimplantation mouse blastocysts (31) which makes biochemical analysis more feasible. Expression of MT genes in the rabbit blastocyst was analyzed by northern blot hybridization with a mouse MT-I cRNA probe. The day-6 rabbit blastocysts contained readily detectable levels of MT-I mRNA (Figure 1; tracks 2 & 4). RNA from day-6 blastocysts incubated *in vitro* with zinc (400 μM) contained significantly increased (about 5-fold) levels of MT-I mRNA (Figure 1; track 5), whereas 40 μM zinc, had little effect (Figure 1; track 3). Incubation of the blastocysts with 10 μM cadmium for 4 h also significantly increased MT-I mRNA levels (Figure 1; track 6). The levels of MT-I mRNA in the blastocyst after incubation for 4 h with 400 μM zinc or 10 μM cadmium approached those found in the zinc-induced adult liver (Fig 1; track 1). Incubation with cadmium resulted in a large induction of HSP-70 mRNA (Figure 1; track 9), whereas zinc had little effect (Figure 1; track 8).

To determine the effects of metal ions on the relative rate of synthesis of MT, blastocysts were cultured with various concentrations of zinc or cadmium, and proteins were subsequently pulse-labeled with ^{35}S-cysteine and labeled cytosolic proteins were carboxymethylated, separated on a 30% polyacrylamide gel (27) and detected by fluorography (Figure 2). Under these conditions, MT has a characteristic mobility which is faster than other cysteine rich proteins in these extracts (1,4,22). Incubation of day-6 blastocysts with zinc resulted in a concentration dependent increase in the relative rate of MT synthesis with a maximal response at between 300 and 600 μM zinc (Figure 2A; tracks 2, 3 & 6). The relative rate of MT synthesis was also increased following incubation with 10 μM cadmium (Figure 2A; track 5), however the magnitude of this induction was much reduced relative to the maximal induction of MT synthesis by zinc (Fig 2A; compare tracks 5 & 6). Incubation of day-4 embryos with 400 μM zinc for 4 h also increased the relative rate of MT synthesis (Figure 2B). About 30% of the day-4 embryos were at the preblastocyst stage of development and 70% were blastocysts.

The above results establish that *in vitro* exposure of rabbit blastocysts to zinc increases the abundance of MT mRNA leading to an increase in the relative rate of MT synthesis. Further analysis established that, in the rabbit blastocyst, both MT-I and -II are induced by metal ions (4). In recent experiments the *in situ* hybridization was used to analyze metallothionein mRNA levels in the day-1 to -4 mouse embryo. The data suggest that the MT genes first become competent to respond to zinc or cadmium at the morula to blastocyst stage of development. Both trophectoderm and inner cell mass could be induced by zinc (Andrews, *et al.,* in press).

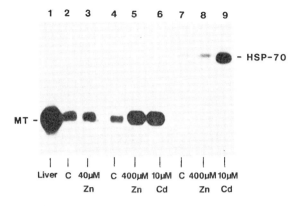

Figure 1. Northern blot detection of MT and HSP-70 in day-6 rabbit blastocysts. RNA (6 µg) was separated on 1.5% agarose-formaldehyde gels and northern blotted to nitrocellulose filters (4,15). Filters were hybridized, under conditions described previously (2), with a ^{32}P-labeled MT-I cRNA probe or with a mouse HSP-70 cRNA probe. After hybridization the filters were washed at 66^0 under stringent conditions and the hybrids were detected by autoradiography. Samples were as follows: Control day-6 blastocysts (C,tracks 2, 4 & 7): Blastocysts incubated for 4 h with 40 µM zinc chloride (track 3); 400 µM zinc chloride (tracks 5 & 8); 10 µM cadmium chloride (tracks 6 & 9): Adult liver after injection of zinc chloride (25 mg/kg, injected 2X in 24 h) (track 1) [from Andrews (4), with permission].

MT Gene Expression in Decidua, Placentae and Visceral Yolk Sac

The decidua contained high levels of MT-I mRNA on D8 through D10. As the placenta developed and replaced the deciduum, MT-I mRNA levels declined, and by D16 placental MT-I mRNA levels were similar to those found in normal adult liver (Figure 3A). Solution hybridization showed that both MT-I and -II mRNAs were elevated about 12-fold relative to adult liver in decidua, and were coordinately reduced during placental development (Table 1). Thus, both MT-I and MT-II mRNAs were in high abundance in D8 deciduum. During formation and maturation of the placenta, levels of MT-I and MT-II mRNAs declined about 6-fold (Table 1).

The visceral yolk sac contained high levels of MT-I mRNA by D14 (Figure 3B). This expression, which has been reported previously, is restricted to the visceral endoderm (2). During the early stages of embryogenesis (D9), MT-I mRNA levels were low in the visceral yolk sac (Figure 3B) as were MT-II mRNA levels (data not shown). These results establish that the mouse MT genes are coordinately expressed in a tissue-specific and temporal manner during gestation: first in the decidua, and later in the placentae and visceral endoderm.

To determine whether synthesis of MT occurs in the decidua and placentae, pulse-labelled proteins from tissue explants were analyzed by polyacrylamide gel electrophoresis (Figure 4). Decidua and placentae were active in the synthesis of a small cysteine-rich, heat-stable protein which comigrated with authentic carboxymethylated MT. These results establish that MT mRNA is actively translated in decidua and placentae. However, the relative rate of synthesis of MT remained high in the D14 placenta despite the decline in MT mRNA levels in total RNA at this stage.

Cell Type-Specific MT Gene Expression in Decidua and Placentae

In situ hybridization was used to examine the cellular distribution of MT-I mRNA during decidual and placental development (Figs. 5 and 6). A variety of controls, including hybridization with sense strand probes, were used to validate this approach (15). MT-I mRNA levels, detected by northern blot hybridization, were very low in the uterus from D1 to 4, but increased soon after implantation (data not shown). MT-I mRNA was localized on

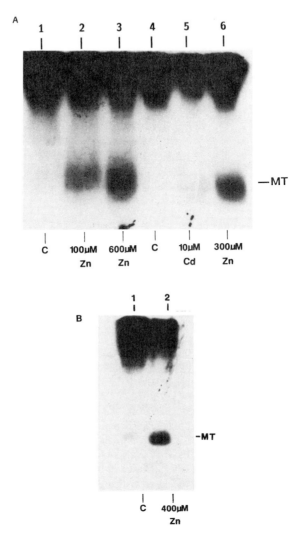

Figure 2. Effects of metal ions on the relative rate of MT synthesis in rabbit blastocysts. **Part A**: day-6 blastocysts were incubated with $ZnCl_2$ or $CdCl_2$ for 5 h and proteins were pulse-labeled with ^{35}S-cysteine during the last hour of culture. Labeled proteins (100,000 cpm) were carboxymethylated, separated by 30% SDS-polyacrylamide gel electrophoresis and detected by fluorography (2,4). Samples were as follows: Controls (C,tracks 1 & 4): 100 μM Zn (track 2); 600 μM Zn (track 3); 10 μM Cd (track 5); and 300 μM Zn (track 6). **Part B**: day-4 rabbit blastocysts were incubated with 400 μM Zn for 4 h and the relative rate of synthesis of MT analyzed as detailed above. The electrophoretic migration of purified rabbit MT is indicated. The isoforms of MT co-migrated in these gels [from Andrews (4), with permission].

Table 1. Metallothionein-I and -II mRNA Levels in Decidua and Placentae during Gestation

Age[a]	MT Isoform[b] I	II
8	11.0	13.4
10	10.0	8.9
12	4.6	4.9
14	3.0	2.2
16	2.0	N.D

[a]Age refers to day of gestation.

[b]Data represent fold-increase in MT-I and MT-II mRNA levels relative to those in control adult liver, as determined by oligodeoxyribonucleotide excess solution hybridization. Liver RNA, obtained 5 h following injection of 100 μmol/kg of $ZnCl_2$ contained 43.0-and 23.0-fold more MT-I and MT-II mRNA than control liver, respectively. Deciduum (D8), deciduum/placenta (D10) and placentae (D12 to 16) were obtained from the conceptuses from 3 to 6 pregnant females, and the results represent the average of three determinations. N.D. means not determined [from De et al.,(15), with permission].

D4 in the uterine luminal epithelium, but was present at relatively low levels (Figure 5, Part A). However, MT-I mRNA was specifically elevated in the primary decidual zone at the site of blastocyst implantation on D5. (Figure 5, Part B). MT-I mRNA was down-regulated in the primary decidua (Figure 5, Part B; DAY 6B), and upregulated in the secondary decidual zone on D6. By D8, MT-I mRNA was located in the peripheral secondary decidual zone (Figure 5, Part B). No hybridization was detected using the sense strand MT probe (Figure 5, Part C).

In situ hybridization demonstrated that spongiotrophoblasts, which are located in the outer placenta, constitutively express high levels of this mRNA (Figure 6). In contrast, the trophoblast giant cells (outer placenta), and labyrinthine trophoblasts (inner placenta) contained little MT-I mRNA. The trophoblast giant cells, however, contained placental lactogen-II mRNA (18) (Figure 6, DAY 12b), and these cells are a major source of synthesis of placental lactogens (30). The demarcation between the high level of MT-I mRNA in the spongiotrophoblasts, and the low level of this mRNA in the labyrinthine trophoblasts on D14 is striking (Figure 6; DAY 14, control). The relative difference in MT-I gene expression between the spongiotrophoblasts and the labyrinthine trophoblasts was maintained following injection of metal. Metal ions induced MT-I mRNA to extremely high levels in the spongiotrophoblasts, and increased the basal levels found in the labyrinthine trophoblasts (Figure 6; DAY 14, zinc-treated). These results establish that MT-I gene expression is regulated in a cell-and temporal-specific manner during formation and maturation of the mouse deciduum and placenta.

Analysis of Regulation of Expression of MT Genes in Mouse Decidua

Currently, several experimental approaches have been applied toward elucidation of the mechanisms which regulate decidual MT genes. In order to examine the involvement of the embryo, the decidual reaction was induced by injection of sesame oil into the utero-tubular junction of pseudopregnant mice on D4. The deciduomata on D8 was then compared with the normal D8 decidua, and no differences in the levels of MT mRNA were noted (15). Therefore, it is apparent that decidual MT gene expression is not dependent on the presence of the embryo or some embryo-derived factor.

The observation that MT mRNA levels in the D8 deciduum are much greater than those in the maternal liver (Fig 3A) suggests a local rather than systemic modulator of MT genes in decidua. The competence of the D4 pregnant uterus to respond to metal ions or cytokines, and the effects of adrenalectomy on decidual MT mRNA were determined, and these data will be published elsewhere (15, De *et al.,* in press). However, in summary, it was found that injection of zinc resulted in only a slight increase in MT mRNA levels in the D4 uterus, whereas maternal liver levels were maximally stimulated. This suggests that the D4 uterus is not exceptionally responsive to zinc, and therefore systemic changes in metal ion levels do not account for elevated decidual MT mRNA levels. Adrenalectomy on D4 did not effect MT mRNA levels in decidua on D8, indicating that glucocorticoids do not play a significant role in decidual MT expression. Furthermore, the treatment of ovariectomized mice with progesterone and/or estrogen had little effect on MT mRNA levels in the uterus. In contrast, an injection of bacterial endotoxin or human recombinant interleukin-1α (IL-1α) or IL-1β rapidly elevated MT mRNA levels several-fold in the D4 uterus. Following injection of endotoxin or IL-1α or β, rapid induction of mRNAs for a variety of cytokines [i.e. IL-1α and β, IL-6, tumor necrosis factor-α (TNF-α)] occurred in the D4 uterus. These results established that exogenous cytokines can enhance MT gene expression in the uterus, and that several cytokine genes in this organ can be upregulated. Northern blot analysis demonstrated the low levels of IL-1α, β and TNF-α mRNAs in the mouse decidua. These results led us to hypothesize that the expression of the decidual MT genes in the mouse is regulated in response to the pro-inflammatory process of implantation and decidualization.

Discussion

MTs are cysteine rich, heavy metal binding proteins (21,28,38) which are known to be expressed in the fetal and neonatal liver (48), and in the visceral endoderm of the developing mouse conceptus (2). The purpose of the studies reported here was to examine the expression and regulation of metallothionein genes from the time of fertilization to midgestation. The preimplantation rabbit and mouse embryos were found to constitutively express low levels of MT at the morula to blastocyst stage of development, and this expression could be dramatically upregulated in response to a short exposure to metal ions in the culture medium. Although the expression of MT genes in the early embryo is low, the finding of elevated expression of the mouse MT genes specifically in decidua and placentae strengthens the concept that MT plays an important role in mammalian embryonic development. Thus, from the time of implantation to late in gestation, the embryo is surrounded by cells which actively express the MT genes: first, the deciduum, and then the spongiotrophoblasts of the placenta, and the visceral yolk sac endoderm. These cell types are each positioned between the maternal and embryonic environments. Therefore, expression of the MT genes is tightly controlled and occurs in a cell-specific and temporally regulated manner during pregnancy.

The functional roles of MT in development are not understood. Elevated MT in the cells surrounding the developing embryo could provide for a local increase in the levels of zinc or copper ions by sequestering them from the maternal serum, and thereby facilitate the rapid growth and differentiation of the embryo. Alternatively, MT may serve to scavenge free radicals (45), and thus protect cells from the injurious effect of these molecules. In this regard, it has been reported that during blastocyst formation in the rabbit, the consumption of oxygen increases 3- to 4-fold (10) which could lead to increased formation of free radicals. The discovery of elevated expression of MT genes in decidua and placentae provides a plausible explanation for the mechanism by which cadmium is rapidly sequestered in these structures. Studies of metal deposition in the embryo and fetus demonstrate that cadmium is almost totally prevented from reaching the embryo (17), and accumulates in the placenta-yolk sac. This suggests that MT may play a protective role during embryogenesis. These results clearly establish that the blastocyst can respond to alterations in environmental metal ion concentration by increased expression of MT genes. During sea urchin development, MT is a maternal mRNA with embryonic MT mRNA synthesis beginning at the 8-cell cleavage

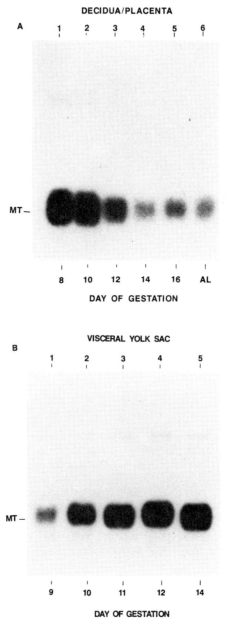

Figure 3. MT-I mRNA levels in mouse decidua, placentae and visceral yolk sacs. RNA was extracted from decidua or placentae (**Part A**), and visceral yolk sacs (**Part B**) on the indicated days of gestation (D1 = vaginal plug). Total RNA (6 µg) was fractionated by formaldehyde-1.5% agarose gel electrophoresis, and analyzed by northern blot hybridization using a mouse MT-I cRNA probe. In **Part A** samples were as follows: lane 1, D8 deciduum; lane 2, D10 deciduum/placenta; lane 3, D12 placenta; lane 4, D14 placenta; lane 5, D16 placenta. For comparative purposes, normal adult liver (lane 6, AL) total RNA, which contains basal levels of MT mRNA, was also analyzed by northern blotting. In all experiments duplicate gels were stained with acridine orange to ensure integrity of the RNA sample and to confirm that equal amounts of RNA had been loaded onto each lane [from De (15) *et al.*, with permission].

71

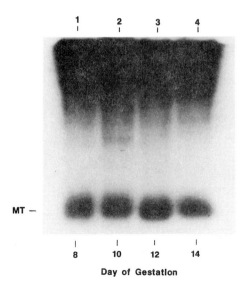

MT —

Day of Gestation

Figure 4. MT synthesis in mouse decidua and placentae. Explants of decidua and placentae were pulse-labeled with ^{35}S-cysteine. Soluble proteins were carboxymethylated, and the heat-stable proteins (80,000 cpm) separated by 20% native polyacrylamide gel electrophoresis and detected by fluorography (22). Samples were as follows: lane 1, D8 deciduum; lane 2, D10 deciduum/placenta; lane 3, D12 placenta; lane 4, D14 placenta. The electrophoretic migration of purified carboxymethylated rat MT is indicated. The isoforms of MT migrated very near each other in these gels [from De et al., (15), with permission].

stage (34). The cell type(s) expressing the MT gene in the rabbit blastocyst has not been identified directly; however, at this stage of development over 90% of the cells are trophoblast cells (31). This makes it likely that these cells are the major source of MT in rabbit blastocysts. Using in situ hybridization it was established that MT genes are constitutively expressed, as well as induced by metal ions, in essentially every cell in the blastocyst and late morula in the mouse (Andrews, in press). The only other inducible gene which has been analyzed for regulation of expression in the mammalian preimplantation embryo is the HSP-70 gene. HSP-70 is inducible by elevated temperature at the blastocyst stage of development in the mouse and rabbit, but not in cleavage stage embryos (24). As reported here, cadmium, which is toxic to the embryo, can also induce HSP-70 in the rabbit blastocyst. Therefore, in the mouse embryo, both of these inducible genes (MT and HSP-70) develop competence to respond to environmental signals at the late morula to blastocyst stage. It has been shown, however, that MT-fusion genes microinjected into the fertilized mouse egg are responsive to metal ions (11). This suggests that the factors necessary for metal ion enhancement of MT gene promoter activity are functional at this stage of development, but that other factors, such as the chromatin structure of the endogenous MT genes, may preclude their induction by metals until the cleavage stages are completed.

The finding of elevated MT mRNA in decidua is unique. The clear demarcation between MT mRNA containing cells in primary decidua on D5, and subsequently in secondary decidua (D6-8), and other uterine cell types, suggests that MT gene expression provides a novel phenotypic marker for murine decidual cells. This may provide a useful tool for analysis of the regulation of decidual cell growth and differentiation. The observation that hepatic expression of MT is dramatically elevated in response to bacterial

A

DAY 4

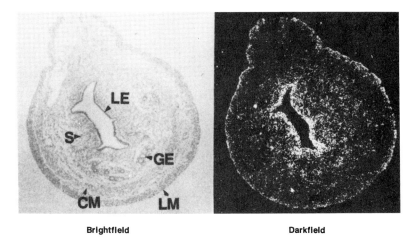

Brightfield   Darkfield

Figure 5. Localization of MT-I mRNA in mouse decidua using *in situ* hybridization. Pregnant mice, on the indicated days of gestation were anesthetized, and tissues were fixed by perfusion with 4% paraformaldehyde in PBS. Samples were paraffin embedded and serially sectioned at 7 μm. MT-I mRNA was hybridized *in situ* for 5 h at 42° with a ^{35}S-labeled MT-I cRNA probe and RNase A resistant hybrids were detected following 4 days of autoradiography using Kodak NTB-2 liquid emulsion. Slides were post-stained lightly in hematoxylin. **Part A:** Brightfield and darkfield photomicrographs (magnification is 40X) of a section of the D4 uterus. Abbreviations are as follows: LE, luminal epithelium; GE, glandular epithelium; CM, circular muscle; LM, longitudinal muscle. **Part B:** Shown here are dark field photomicrographs of sections of decidua which were hybridized on the same microscope slide. Magnification is 40X, except for day 6B which is 100X. PDZ; primary decidual zone; SDZ; secondary decidual zone. **Part C:** Darkfield photomicrographs (magnification is 40X) of sections of the D7 deciduum after *in situ* hybridization with antisense or sense strand MT probes [from De *et al.*, (15), with permission].

infection, an effect mediated by endotoxin (35), has lead to the classification of MT as an acute-phase protein (29). In this regard, it has recently been reported that the rat decidua synthesizes two other major acute phase proteins, α(1)-acid glycoprotein (44) and α(2)-macroglobulin (20). This suggests that a primary function of the decidua may be related to the protective roles these proteins play in response to stress. These results also suggest a common mechanism of regulation of these genes in the decidua (see below). With regard to placental MT, others have reported MT-like proteins in human (47) and rat placentae (12), and cadmium induces MT protein in mouse and rat placentae (48).

What regulates decidual and placental MT gene expression is under investigation in this laboratory. Maternal systemic effects have been suggested to influence hepatic MT expression in the fetus. Glucocorticoids increase in the maternal circulation most dramatically after D10 gestation (7), and appear to enhance both maternal and fetal hepatic MT gene expression in the mouse (39). Maternal dietary zinc deficiency causes reduced hepatic MT mRNA levels in the newborn rat (3) and mouse (46). Studies in this laboratory (15), suggest that elevated expression of decidual MT (D8) does not involve either elevated zinc or glucocorticoids in the maternal serum, but rather a local effect may be mediating expression of these genes. Analysis of MT gene expression in artificially induced deciduomata suggests that in decidua, this expression does not require the presence of the embryo or some embryo derived factor (15). However, several lines of evidence suggest that locally released cytokines may be involved in regulation of decidual MT genes. An injection of bacterial endotoxin or

B

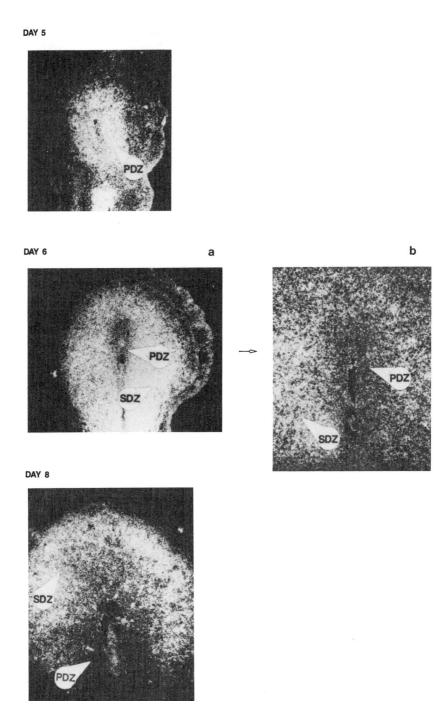

DAY 5

PDZ

DAY 6   a   b

PDZ

SDZ

PDZ

SDZ

DAY 8

SDZ

PDZ

Figure 5B (see legend for 5A).

C

Antisense Probe   Sense Probe

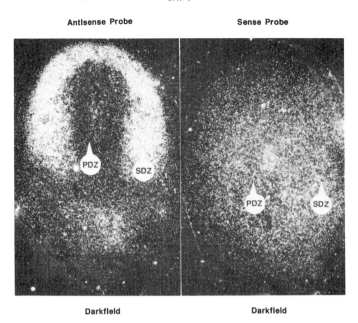

Darkfield   Darkfield

Figure 5C (see legend for 5A).

recombinant cytokines (IL-1α or β) induces MT mRNA in the uterus on D4 of gestation just prior to implantation. This establishes that just before implantation the MT genes in the uterus are competent to respond to these factors. The mRNAs for several cytokines are present in low levels in the decidua, and the levels of these mRNAs can be upregulated by endotoxin. These observations could serve to explain the common expression of several acute phase protein genes in the decidua.

The suggestion of the possible importance of various cytokines and lymphokines in the physiology of pregnancy is not unique to our studies of MT regulation in the decidua, but has received much recent attention. Macrophages have been identified near the site of embryo implantation (43), and the production of interleukins by the rabbit uterine cervix (26), and by freshly explanted human endometrial cells (42) has been described. IL-1 can stimulate chorionic gonadotropin release from human placental trophoblast (49), and IL-2 is expressed by human placental syncytiotrophoblast (9). Therefore, it seems likely that a variety of important processes during pregnancy are mediated by the local production of such factors by the uterus, decidua and placenta. The cell-types responsible for the synthesis of these cytokines remains to be determined.

In summary, our evidence suggests that the MT genes become competent to respond to increased concentrations of zinc and cadmium in the environment at about the blastocyst stage of development. Following implantation, specific cells which are interposed between the fetal and maternal environments (decidua, placental spongiotrophoblasts, visceral yolk sac endoderm) display heightened expression of MT. This suggests that MT may play an important role in the establishment and maintenance of normal pregnancy.

DAY 12

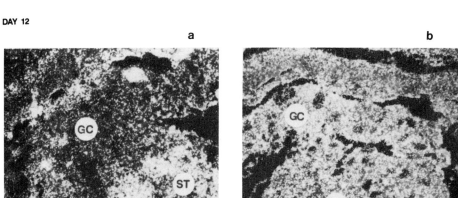

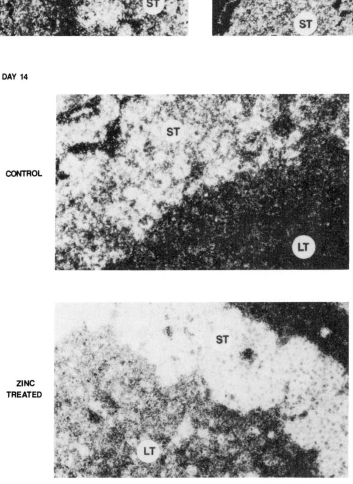

Figure 6. Localization of MT-I mRNA in mouse placentae by *in situ* hybridization. Placentae, on the indicated days of gestation, were analyzed by *in situ* hybridization as described in the legend to Figure 5. Autoradiography was for 4 days (sections were on the same slide), and slides were post-stained lightly with hematoxylin. Shown here are dark field photomicrographs (40X magnification) of longitudinal sections near the outer edge through the mid-region of placentae. Day-12a, MT-I mRNA localization; GC, giant trophoblast cells; ST, spongiotrophoblast cells. Day-12b, placental lactogen-II mRNA localization. Day-14; MT-I mRNA localization; ST, spongiotrophoblast; LT, labyrinthine trophoblast; zinc-treated, placenta taken 4 h following injection of 100 μmol zinc/kg body weight [from De *et al.*, (15), with permission].

Acknowledgments

We wish to thank Drs. Yvette Huet-Hudson and Lois Lehman-McKeenan, and Shelly Shepard, and Joanne Orth for assistance in these experiments. This work was supported (in part) by BRSG S07 RR05373 awarded by the Biomedical Research Support Grant Program, Division of Research Resources and by grants from the NIH (ES 04725) to G. K. Andrews, and (HD 12304) to S. K. Dey. S. K. De is funded by the Wesley Foundation Scholar Program in Cancer Research postdoctoral fellowship. M. T. McMaster is a March of Dimes predoctoral fellow.

References

1. Andersen, R. D., Piletz, J. E., Birren, B. W., and Herschman, H. R., Levels of metallothionein in fetal, neonatal and maternal rat liver. Eur. J. Biochem. 131:497 (1983).
2. Andrews, G. K., Adamson, E. D., and Gedamu, L., The ontogeny of expression of murine metallothionein: comparison with the α-fetoprotein gene. Dev. Biol. 103:294 (1984).
3. Andrews, G. K., Gallant, K. R., and Cherian, M. G., Regulation of the ontogeny of rat liver metallothionein by zinc. Eur. J. Biochem. 166:527 (1987).
4. Andrews, G. K., Lehman, L. D., Huet, Y. M., and Dey. S. K., Metallothionein gene regulation in the preimplantation rabbit blastocyst. Development, 100:463 (1987).
5. Angerer, L. M. and Angerer, R. C., Detection of poly-A+ RNA in sea urchin eggs and embryos by quantitative in situ hybridization. Nucl. Acids Res. 9:2819 (1981).
6. Angerer, L. M., Deleon, D. V., Angerer, R. C., Showman, R. M., Wells, D. E., and Raff, R. A., Delayed accumulation of maternal histone mRNA during sea urchin oogenesis. Dev. Biol. 101:477 (1984).
7. Barlow, S. M., Morrison, P. J., and Sullivan, F. M., Plasma corticosterone levels during pregnancy in the mouse: the relative contributions of the adrenal glands and the feto-placental units. J. Endocr. 60:473 (1974).
8. Barlow, S. M. and Sullivan, F. M., Cadmium and its compounds. In: *Reproductive Hazards of Industrial Chemicals.* Barlow, S. M. and Sullivan, F. M. (eds.), London: Academic Press, p. 136 (1982).
9. Boehm, K. D., Kelley, M. F., Ilan, J., and Ilan, J., The interleukin-2 gene is expressed in the syncytiotrophoblast of the human placenta. Proc. Natl. Acad. Sci. USA 86:656 (1989).
10. Brinster, R. L., Embryo development. J. Animal Sci. 38:1003 (1974).
11. Brinster, R. L., Chen, H. Y., Warren, R., Sarthy, A., and Palmiter, R. D., Regulation of metallothionein-thymidine kinase fusion plasmids injected into mouse eggs. Nature 296:39 (1982).
12. Charles-Shannon, V. L., Sasser, L. B., Burbank, D. K., and Kelman, B. L., The influence of zinc on the ontogeny of hepatic metallothionein in the fetal rat. Proc. Soc. Exper. Biol. Med. 168:56 (1981).
13. Cousins, R. J., Toward a molecular understanding of zinc metabolism. Clin. Physiol. Biochem. 4:20 (1986).
14. Cox, K. H., Deleon, D. V., Angerer, L. M., and Angerer, R. C., Detection of mRNAs in sea urchin embryos by in situ hybridization using asymmetric RNA probes. Dev. Biol. 101:485 (1984).
15. De, S. K., McMaster, M. T., Dey, S. K., and Andrews, G. K., Cell-specific metallothionein gene expression in mouse decidua and placentae. Development, 107:611 (1989).

16. Deleon, D. V., Cox, K. H., Angerer, L. M., and Angerer, R. C., Most early-variant histone mRNA is contained in the pronucleus of sea urchin eggs. Dev. Biol. 100:197 (1983).

17. Dencker, L., Danielsson, B., Khayat, A., and Lindgren, A., Disposition of metals in the embryo and fetus. In: *Reproductive and Developmental Toxicity of Metals*. Clarkson, T. W., Nordberg, G. F., and Sager, P. R. (eds.), New York, Plenum Press, pp. 607-631. (1983).

18. Duckworth, M. L., Peden, L. M., and Friesen, H. G., Isolation of a novel prolactin-like cDNA clone from developing rat placenta. J. Biol. Chem. 261:10879 (1986).

19. Durnam, D. M. and Palmiter, R. D., A practical approach for quantitating specific mRNAs by solution hybridization. Anal. Biochem. 131:385 (1983).

20. Fletcher, S., Thomas, T., Schreiber, G., Heinrich, P. C., and Yeoh, G. C. T., The development of rat α_2-macroglobulin. Eur. J. Biochem 171:703 (1988).

21. Hamer, D. H., Metallothioneins. Ann. Rev. Biochem. 55:913 (1986).

22. Hamer, D. J. and Walling, M., Regulation *in vivo* of a cloned mammalian gene: cadmium induces transcription of a mouse metallothionein gene in SV40 vectors. J. Mol. Appl. Genet. 1:273 (1982) .

23. Hayashi, S., Gillam, I. C., Delaney, A. D., and Tener, G. M., Acetylation of chromosome squashes of Drosophila melanogaster decreases the background in autoradiographs from hybridization with [^{125}I]-labeled RNA J. Histochem. Cytochem. 26:677 (1978).

24. Heikkila, J. J., Miller, J. O., Schultz, G. A., Kloc, M., and Browder, L., Heat shock expression during early animal development. In: *Changes in Gene Expression in Response to Environmental Stress*. Atkinson, B. G. and Walden, D. B., (eds.), New York, Academic Press, pp. 135-158. (1985).

25. Hurley, L. S. and Shrader, R. E., Abnormal development of preimplantation rat eggs after three days of maternal dietary zinc deficiency. Nature 254:427 (1975).

26. Ito, A., Hiro, D., Oijma, Y., and Mori, Y., Spontaneous production of interleukin-1-like factors from the rabbit uterine cervix. Am. J. Obstet. Gynecol. 159:261 (1988).

27. Kagi, J. H. R. and Schaffer, A., Biochemistry of metallothionein. Biochemistry 27:8509 (1988).

28. Karin, M., Metallothioneins: proteins in search of function. Cell. 41:9 (1985).

29. Koj, A. In: *The Acute Phase Response to Injury and Infection*. Gordon, A. H. and Kol, A. (eds.), Elsevier, Amsterdam, chapter 13 (1985).

30. Lee, S. J., Talamantes, F., Wilder, E., Linzer, D. I. H., and Nathans, D., Trophoblastic giant cells of the mouse placenta as the site of proliferin synthesis. Endocrinology 122:1761 (1988).

31. Lutwak-Mann, C., Some physiological and biochemical properties of the mammalian blastocyst. Bull. Swiss. Acad. Med. Sci. 22:101 (1966).

32. Melton, D. A., Krieg, P. A., Rebegliati, M. R., Maniatis, T., Kinn, K., and Green, M. R., Efficient *in vitro* synthesis of biologically active RNA and RNA hybridization probes from plasmids containing a bacteriophage SP6 promoter. Nucl. Acids. Res. 12:7035 (1984).

33. Mukherjee, A., Dey, S. K., Sengupta, J., Ramadoss, C. S., and Dickmann, Z., Regulatory enzymes of carbohydrate and energy metabolism in the rabbit blastocyst. J. Reprod. Fert. 53:77 (1978).

34. Nemer, M., Travaglini, E. C., Rondinelli, E., and D'Alonzo, J., Developmental regulation, induction, and embryonic tissue specificity of sea urchin metallothionein gene expression. Dev. Biol. 102:471 (1984).

35. Oh, S. H., Deagen, J. T., Whanger, P. D., and Weswig, P. H., Biological function of metallothionein V. Its induction in rats by various stresses. Am. J. Physiol. 234:E282 (1978).

36. Omiecinski, C. J., Walz, F. G., and Vlasuk, G. P., Phenobarbital induction of rat liver cytochromes p-450b and p-450e: quantitation of specific RNAs by hybridization to synthetic oligodeoxyribonucleotide probes. J. Biol. Chem. 260:3247 (1985).

37. Pakrasi, P. L. and Dey, S. K., Catechol estrogens stimulate synthesis of prostaglandins in the preimplantation rabbit blastocyst and endometrium. Biol. Reprod. 29:347 (1983).

38. Palmiter, R. D., Molecular biology of metallothionein gene expression. Experientia (Suppl.) 52:63 (1987).
39. Quaife, C., Hammer, R. E., Mottet, N. K., and Palmiter, R. D., Glucocorticoid regulation of metallothionein during embryonic development. Dev. Biol. 118:549 (1986).
40. Rogers, J.M. and Hurley, L. S., Effects of zinc deficiency on morphogenesis of the fetal rat eye. Development, 99:231 (1987).
41. Searle, P. F., Davison, B. L., Stuart, G. W., Wilkie, T. M., Norstedt, G., and Palmiter, R. D., Regulation, linkage and sequence of mouse metallothionein-I and II genes. Mol. Cell. Biol. 4:1221 (1984).
42. Tabibzadeh, S. S., Santhanam, U., Sehgal, P. B., and May, L. T., Cytokine induced production of IFN-β_2/IL-6 by freshly explanted human endometrial stromal cells. J. Immunol. 142:3134 (1989).
43. Tachi, C., Tachi, S., Knyszynski, A., and Lindner, H. R., Possible involvement of macrophages in embryo-maternal relationships during ovum implantation in the rat. J. Exptl. Zool. 217:81 (1981).
44. Thomas, T., Fletcher, S., Yeoh, G. C. T., and Schreiber, G., The expression of $\alpha(1)$-acid glycoprotein mRNA during rat development. J. Biol. Chem. 264:5784 (1989).
45. Thornalley, P. J. and Vasak, M., Possible role for metallothionein in protection against radiation-induced oxidative stress. Kinetics and mechanism of its reaction with superoxide and hydroxyl radicals. Biochem. Biophys. Acta. 827:36 (1985).
46. Vruwink, K. G., Hurley, L. S., Gershwin, M. E., and Keen, C. L., Gestational zinc deficiency amplifies the regulation of metallothionein induction in adult mice. Proc. Soc. Exptl. Biol. Med. 188:30 (1988).
47. Waalkes, M. P., Poisner, A. M., Wood, G. W., and Klaassen, C. D., Metallothionein-like proteins in human placenta and fetal membranes. Toxicol. Appl. Pharmacol. 74:179 (1984).
48. Webb, M., Metallothionein in regeneration, reproduction and development. Experi. Suppl. 52:483 (1987).
49. Yagel, S., LaLa, P. K., Powell, W. A., and Casper, R. F., Interleukin-1 stimulates human chorionic gonadotropin secretion by first trimester human trophoblasts. J. Clin. Endocrinol. Metab. 68:992 (1989).
50. Yu, J. S., Tarr, P. P. L., and Chan, S. T. H., Effects of cadmium on preimplantation mouse embryos *in vitro* with special reference to their implantation capacity and subsequent development. Teratology 32:347 (1985).

Questions

Dr. Glasser: Is it possible that the cytokines are localized to lymphocytes or macrophages?

Dr. Andrews: I think that it is entirely possible. Tachi & Tachi have recently published a paper which indicates the localization we see for TNF*a* is almost the same as that for macrophages in the decidua. Gary Wood's lab has also shown similar things; they have a poster on this at this conference. But we can't conclude from these studies that macrophages are the sole source of these cytokines. It's clear that a variety of cell types such as fibroblasts and endothelia can make cytokines.

Dr. Glasser: We found that in looking at the late secretory phase of the menstrual cycle-stromal cells undergo what Noyes termed as a predicual cell. These cells decidualize without a blastocyst signal. These might be interesting in terms of an inflammatory response, as perhaps other models might.

Dr. Andrews: The next step is to show more directly, by *in vitro* studies, that we can regulate decidual cell gene expression by cytokines. On the other hand, how you rid that preparation of macrophages is not clear to me. Even how you recognize macrophages is not clear. Lala's group would argue that a variety of these decidual cells are of hematopoetic origin. They may the cells producing cytokines. It's a bit of a bag of worms, for sure. There are a variety of genes now, acute phase proteins which are made in the liver in response to an inflammatory stimulus. In the last six months three of these other genes, in addition to metallothionein shown here, have been localized in the rat decidua. These include alpha-2-macroglobulin, acid-1-glycoprotein, ceruloplasmin. These are induced and regulated by cytokines and found in the decidua.

Dr. Larson: What kind of specificity does metallothionein show in terms of metals? Do they bind to all kinds of metals?

Dr. Andrews: They bind to many transition state metals. Physiologically, they bind to zinc and copper. When zinc binds, it's in equilibrium, and the off reaction is very fast. So it can give up the zinc, even though it binds with high affinity. The dissociation constant is 10^{-12} molar. It's not an irreversible binding. Cadmium, on the other hand, binds and stays bound. So that's one way that you can envision that metallothionein and the decidua can combine to prevent cadmium from traversing that barrier, whereas zinc can actually build up in that locale and, by equilibrium, provide the embryo with the zinc it needs to develop very rapidly.

Dr. Larson: How about iron, does it bind?

Dr. Andrews: Very, very, poorly.

Dr. Glasser: How about zinc deficiencies, what effect does that have?

Dr. Andrews: We've done a lot of work on zinc deficiency. It's a difficult problem. During early development, zinc deficiency terminates pregnancy. We've looked at what may regulate metallothionein in the liver, which in the fetus, is the major source of rat synthesis. Zinc deficiency clearly down-regulates metallothionein. But in the decidua it's a hard problem to touch.

Dr. Dey: If interleukins increase after fertilization what is the response to that on days one, two or three of metallothionein synthesis?

Dr. Andrews: Some of the work which has been done in Gary Wood's lab and my lab shows that interleukins are very high on the first days of pregnancy and they decrease abruptly on days 3 to 4. We thought, if that's true, why isn't metallothionein high on day one and two? In fact, the uterus develops the competence to respond to endotoxin, and on days 1 and 2, if you give an exogenous stimulus like LPS (lipopolysaccharide) you can induce only minimal amounts of metallothionein mRNA in the uterus. That capacity increases and is maximal by day 4. This may be a desensitization, or perhpaps it reflects development of the predecidual cell; maybe metallothionein can provide a marker for that process.

Dr. Dey: How do estrogen and progesterone affect the level of metallothionein message?

Dr. Andrews: We know from some work that we did that combinations of estrogens and progesterone don't effect the level of metallothionein message in the uterus. So we can eliminate them as sources of regulating this gene.

7

Uterine Preparation for Blastocyst Attachment

Joy Mulholland and Stanley R. Glasser
Department of Cell Biology
Center for Population Research and Studies in Reproductive Biology
Baylor College of Medicine
Houston, Texas 77030

Summary

Existing models used to analyze uterine receptivity to blastocyst attachment have thus far failed to account for non-genotypic embryonic loss following *in vitro* fertilization and embryo transfer in any species. Although application of the technology for biochemistry and molecular biology has yielded useful information about the uterus at a molecular level, the regulatory mechanisms of ovoreceptivity and implantation remain elusive.

Separation of the component uterine cell types has demonstrated that uterine epithelial and stromal cells can respond independently as well as interdependently to the same regulatory signal. Biochemical and immunocytochemical analysis of these responses can be extended further by development of *in vitro* culture systems which resemble as closely as possible the conditions of cellular growth and development *in vivo*.

Such an *in vitro* culture system has been developed for primary cultures of uterine epithelial cells. When grown on EHS matrix-coated semi-permeable filters, the cells attach, proliferate to confluence and establish morphological and functional indices of polarity. Uterine epithelial cells cultured under these conditions demonstrate a basal preference for amino acid uptake, are active in both apical and basal secretion, and are responsive to steroid hormones. When blastocysts are co-cultured with estrogen-treated epithelial cells, they fail to attach. These same embryos attach readily, however, if transferred to matrix-coated filters, plastic culture wells, or cultures of uterine stromal cells. The polarized epithelial cell culture therefore appears to provide a functional *in vitro* model for ovoreceptivity and embryo attachment.

Introduction

The concept of ovoreceptivity was derived almost 20 years ago from studies using the technique of embryo transfer (41). By definition it is the condition, unique and exclusive to the uterus, which allows blastocyst attachment to occur. Receptivity represents the cooperativity, first recognized by M.C. Chang, between the embryo and the uterus and is delimited by the chronological relationship, i.e., synchrony, between the age of the embryos and the developmental stages of the endometrial cell types (7,36). These developmental relationships are not equally as strict in all species. In some species, e.g., rat and mouse, the blastocyst can wait for the uterus to acquire receptivity (34,36). In other species such as sheep, embryos younger than the uterus can be developmentally accelerated to synchronize with endometrial development (2). Manipulation of the limits of synchrony operate under constraints. For each species, intrauterine survival of transferred embryos, at any stage, cannot be supported beyond the transient phase of uterine receptivity, as the uterus then becomes refractory, entering a stage of non-receptivity (32,39).

Uterine Receptivity: Synchrony versus Asynchrony

The degree of success (implantation, live births) which characterizes embryo transfer in laboratory species (>85%) has not been attained following embryo transfer of human, cow or sheep embryos (44). Most of these losses, elevated still further with transfer of micromanipulated and/or cryopreserved embryos, occur within the first three weeks of pregnancy. It has not yet become feasible to determine statistically whether factors governing embryonic development or factors affecting uterine preparation - or both - are responsible for these early losses. Information covering the earliest periods when the greatest number of embryos are lost is fragmented and conflicting. It is assumed, however, that a significant proportion of embryos are lost for reasons other than genetic imperfection. Extensive studies with farm animals indicate that natural asynchrony is a major cause of embryonic loss (37,55). These studies have defined the limits of uterine tolerance for out-of-phase embryos, but have not provided much information about the developmental stage of the uterus or the causes of embryonic death. Embryos with no genotypic abnormalities may be lost because they fail to develop programmatically. Either they fail to signal their presence to the mother or the signal is not received and/or transduced by the endometrial cells. Thus, asynchronous embryos may die because the uterine luminal environment is only narrowly permissive; it does not always support the normal schedule of growth and development and may even be toxic (35,38). It is evident from continuing attempts to improve the success of IVF/ET programs that the mechanisms regulating the interactions between embryos and the uterine endometrium of any species are little understood. The available data cannot be used predictably to enhance the productivity of these programs.

For economic - as well as ethical and legal - reasons laboratory animals, particularly rodents, have been the primary subjects of research on ovoreceptivity. Species differences related to developmental schedules and dominant hormones are recognized; however, data obtained from rats and mice have been productively extrapolated to other species. The hormonal requirements for uterine receptivity in the rat have been well defined (14,30,40). Ovariectomized animals are used for the analysis of ovoreceptivity which is composed of three phases, described below.

The Prereceptive Phase

A minimum of 48h exposure to progesterone (P, 2-5 mg/d X3) is required to develop a prereceptive uterus which is not hostile to the presence of viable embryos but does not allow blastocyst attachment (39,40). This prereceptive status can be maintained and extended (diapause) by continuous exposure to P, i.e., PX5, PX7 (14,16). The natural homolog of the experimental prereceptive uterus is the preimplantation uterus from 24h after conception (fertilization is considered as to time zero) until 36h after a nidatory surge of estrogen (E) peaks at approximately 60h after conception (54).

The Receptive Phase

A single injection of estradiol-17β (E2) (50 ng) to a PX3 treated rat will initiate the transition from a pre-receptive to receptive uterus (14,20,41). Receptivity is transient, extending over a period of 12-36h following the E2 injection. A receptive uterus will allow blastocysts to attach to the luminal epithelium. Receptive uterine epithelial cells are involved, in some way yet to be defined, in transducing an attachment related signal to the cells of the stromal compartment. Presumably, this signal will induce subsequent differentiation of uterine

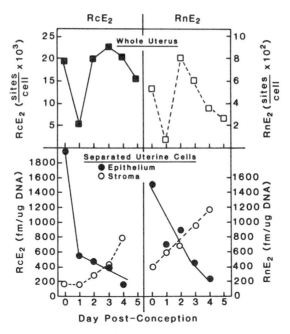

Figure 1. Concentrations of cytoplasmic (R_cE_2) and nuclear (R_nE_2) estrogen receptors in the whole uterus were measured on successive days of gestation following fertilization on day 0 (upper panels). The respective concentrations of R_cE_2 and R_nE_2 were also measured in isolated rat uterine epithelial and stromal cells on different post-conception days (lower panels). When these data were compared with those obtained from whole uterus marked differences in the profile were apparent.

stromal cells (12). The natural homolog of the receptive uterus occurs in the pregnant animal 36-48h following secretion of nidatory E. If attachment fails to occur the cascade of modulated events initiated by nidatory E sequentially effects transformation from a receptive to a refractory uterus.

The Refractory Phase

A refractory uterus will not support blastocyst attachment, will not decidualize, and will not maintain embryos in an active or diapaused condition. Therefore, the refractory uterus is not the endocrinological or physiological equivalent of the prereceptive uterus. Although initiated by nidatory E, the refractory state is maintained by P (16,39). In order for the uterus to return to a neutral status P must be withdrawn for at least 48h (39,40).

Hormone Responses of Separated Endometrial Cell Types

A number of changes or events have been advanced as possible indicators of the receptive uterus. Included on this list is an increase in uterine vascular flux; specifically, a local increase in capillary permeability (39). This type of vascular change infers the delivery and/or removal of signal or repressor molecules. None of these has specifically been identified or correlated with receptivity. Thinning of the apical glycocalyx, reduction in negative cell surface charge, activation of monoamine oxidase and other classes of enzymes, changes in the patterns of luminal protein and glycoprotein secretion and shifting profiles of

Table 1. The use of separated endometrial cells vs. whole uterus for the study of biochemical mechanisms regulating implantation: Advantages and limitations

Separated Cells	Whole Uterus
1. Responses are cell specific. Can distinguish between populations of resident cells in each compartment of endometrium.	1. Data represents net responses (not cell specific).
2. Responses are stage-specific.	2. Responses may be stage specific.
3. Responses are factor specific.	3. Responses may be factor specific.
4. Mechanistic analysis can be done on individual cells or cell-cell recombinations (synchronous, asynchronous; homotypic, heterotypic).	4. Mechanistic analyses are not practical.
5. Disrupts normal tissue organization. Under certain conditions cell expression may be arrested or altered.	5. Maintains tissue architecture and organization.
6. Limited secreted material from a single cell type.	6. Limited secreted material of uncertain origin.
7. Limited numbers of cells.	7. Limited numbers of cells.

apical lectin binding have all been put forward as characteristics of a receptive uterus (1,41). Practically, it has not been possible to assign a determinative role to any of these changes in terms of uterine receptivity. To some extent this difficulty arises from the use of the whole uterus to measure what are likely to be cell-specific properties. The architecture and cellular heterogeneity of the uterus, even the entire endometrium, are intricate and in constant flux. Important cell-specific responses can be masked by measuring responses in total uterine tissue. In addition all these studies seeking to identify and isolate marker molecules lack an exacting bioassay system which allows a cell-specific and/or stage-specific molecule to be assigned an implantation determinative role.

Pre- and peri-implantation changes have been described in terms of receptor-mediated events that could regulate the biochemical expression describing the receptive uterus. These studies have produced interesting data but analyses of steroid hormone receptors of the whole uterus (Fig. 1) or at sites of implantation have not proven particularly effective in identifying those processes by which the non-receptive uterus is transformed to receptivity (15,27). Experiments citing the separate responses of the continuously changing population of rat endometrial cell types (51) suggested that cell heterogeneity prevented the deduction of cause and effect relationships in the analysis of blastocyst attachment. Cell separation procedures have been developed to overcome this problem (33). Cytoplasmic (R_CE2) and nuclear (R_NE2) estrogen receptor analyses of homogeneous populations of separated rat uterine epithelial and stromal cells (Fig. 1, lower panels) on various days following conception showed that cells in each of the compartments of the endometrium responded independently yet interdependently to the same signals (33). These results are more compatible with the physiological data (51) than receptor analyses of the whole preimplantation rat uterus (Fig. 1, upper panel).

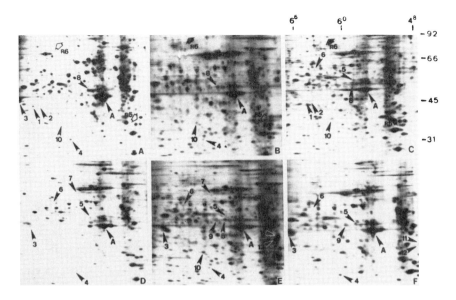

Figure 2. Two dimensional gel electrophoretic profiles of proteins synthesized by uterine epithelial (A-C) and stromal cells (D-F) separated during the prereceptive (A,D), receptive (B,E) and refractory periods of ovoreceptivity. Molecular weight markers are noted in kilodaltons and the pH gradient is marked at the top of 2C. Protein "A" is actin. Specific proteins in both epithelial and stromal cells are numbered and marked with arrowheads. See Mulholland and Leroy (32) for detailed discussion.

In Vitro **Culture of Polarized Primary Uterine Epithelial Cells**

The benefits of using separated cells to study uterine preparation for nidation outbalance the limitations (Table 1), particularly for studies on a cellular or molecular basis. Separated rat endometrial cells have been used to characterize the stages of the peri-implantation uterus. Patterns of protein expression were used to identify stage-specific profiles of uterine epithelial and stromal cell cytosolic proteins (Fig. 2) (32). Fourteen days after ovariectomy rats were made prereceptive by treating them daily for three days with progesterone (PX3, 5 mg). Prereceptive animals were rendered receptive by treating with a single injection of estradiol-17β (E2, 50 ng). Cells were separated and analyzed 16 (receptive) and 40 (refractory) hours after the E2 injection. The transition of prereceptive (PX3; Fig. 2A) to receptive (PX3+E, 16h; Fig 2B) uterine epithelial cells was characterized by the disappearance of three proteins (#1,#2,#3) observed in the prereceptive uterus. No proteins which characterize the receptive uterine epithelial cell appeared to be selectively synthesized, or synthesized *de novo*, by receptive uterine epithelial cells. In contrast, five new proteins (#8,#9,#10,#11,#12) appear in the cells of the uterine stromal compartment during the receptive period (Fig. 2E). The possibility must be considered that these proteins could influence the immediate (receptive) as well as the later (refractory) responses of both the stromal (autocrine) and epithelial (paracrine) cells. In refractory animals two proteins (#5,#6) appear *de novo* in uterine epithelial cells (Fig. 2C) and two proteins (#1,#2) which were repressed during the transition from prereceptive to the receptive phase (Figs. 2A,2B) reappear in the refractory cells. Some proteins (#5,#6,#8) are expressed differentially in stromal or epithelial cells in response to the same hormonal treatment. These experiments confirm previous studies (Fig. 1) because they demonstrate that uterine epithelial and stromal cells respond directly and differentially to the same hormonal signal (32,33).

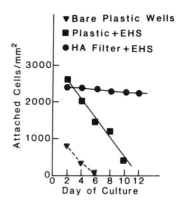

Figure 3. The influence of substratum on proliferation and attachment of uterine epithelial cells separated from immature rats. Not more than 20% of UE cells cultured on bare tissue culture plastic dishes (▼) attach within 24 hours. These UE cells then detach so that none remain by the sixth day. When UE cells are placed onto tissue culture wells covered with EHS-matrix they attach and proliferate to confluence within 48-72 hours (■) (19). These cells do not maintain their confluent density; detachment is complete within 10-12 days. When UE cells are cultured on EHS-matrix covered semi-permeable filters they also attach and proliferate to confluence within 48 hours (●). However they maintain their confluent density and continue to grow (19).

The loss of epithelial protein species also suggests the possibility that receptivity is a repression phenomenon. Earlier experiments which indicated that the mechanisms responsible for receptivity are operable on the level of transcription also showed that these critical events might involve repression or derepression (14). Conversion of the neutral castrate uterus to a prereceptive uterus (PX3) increased the number of transcription initiation sites from 4,000 to 20,000/µg DNA. Surprisingly, and in support of a repressive action (see Fig. 2B) E2 depressed the number of sites to control levels within 4h. These uteri could be decidualized during the 24h which follows E2 treatment after which time they became refractory (14). The relevance of data resulting from short term studies of separated cells suggests that further advances could be gained by extending these methods. Different experimental protocols could integrate the data on cell-associated proteins with expression in the plasma membrane domains and secretory compartments. This would provide a sounder base to analyze factor-directed synthesis and secretion (31,53). Development of *in vitro* cell culture models would provide even further benefits that could be derived from the study of separated cells, particularly if the model provided access to the basal surface of epithelial cells. Current research is being directed towards the development of reliable and reproducible culture methods to define how each cell type responds to a given regulatory factor, or combination of factors (19,20). Protocols have been designed which recognize that *in vivo* both the apical and basal surfaces of UE cells are regulated to function in cell-cell, cell-substratum interactions as well as in absorption, transport and secretion. Historically, these latter properties of the UE cell have been the focus in describing the transition to receptivity.

In Vitro **Implantation**

While short-term incubation studies for analysis of isolated endometrium or endometrial cell types may be considered adequate, the use of long-term protocols (greater than 48-60h) have been the source of much disinformation. Conventional *in vitro* cell culture systems have been less than satisfactory. The utility of such systems, particularly as a model for *in vitro* implantation, has been faulted because they failed to provide a three dimensional

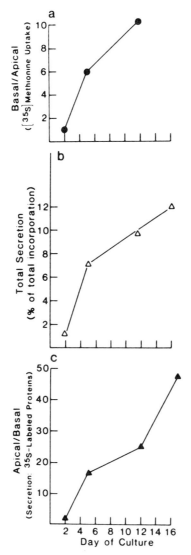

Figure 4. Primary UE cells isolated from immature rats and cultured on EHS-matrix covered semi-permeable filters exhibit functional indices representative of polarity. (a) Development of a basolateral preference for the uptake of [^{35}S]-methionine. Uptake (10 min) was measured from either the apical or basal surface of the filter culture. Data is expressed as the ratio of basal vs. apical uptake of TCA-precipitable cpm incorporated into protein. Studies were conducted on day 2 (preconfluent), day 5 (early confluent) and day 12 (late post-confluent) cultures. (b) Post-confluent UE cells increase their total secretory activity when cultured under these conditions. Total secretion (TCA-precipitable cpm in UE cell apical plus basal secretions) is expressed as the percentage of total TCA-precipitable cpm incorporated into UE cells and their secretions. Cultures were incubated eight hours with [^{35}S]-methionine on culture days 2,5,12 and 16. (c) Polarized UE cells develop an apical preference for secretion. Comparison of TCA-precipitable cpm secreted into the apical relative to that secreted into the basal secretory compartment was made after 8 hours incubation with [^{35}-S]-methionine on day 2,5,12 and 16 of culture (19).

organization typical of tissues *in situ* (10). These conditions are particularly important in the study of simple secretory epithelial cells which must be polarized to express the specialized functions unique to the epithelial cell (49). Since the programmed production of a unique adhesive apical uterine epithelial (UE) surface, either by directed synthesis or derepression,is considered a specialized function of the UE cell, previous culture systems to study UE cells have been limited by their inability to establish cell polarity.

Separation (polarization) of the plasma membrane domains (apical vs. basal-lateral) is obligatory for absorptive, secretory and transporting epithelial cells and cell lines to express their special functions (45,49). Important in this regard is the integrity of intercellular junctions of the lateral paracellular space and their responses to environmental signals (3,42). Secretory epithelial cells from kidney, intestine or liver isolated as single cells attach efficiently (~75%) within 24h and proliferate to confluence within 48h (46,49). Initial studies with separated UE cells showed them to be more difficult to establish in culture. In the presence of culture medium containing 10% fetal calf serum (FCS) only 20% of UE cells from pre-implantation uteri (day 4) or 30% from immature uteri attached to tissue culture plates at 24h. Attachment of UE cells from sexually mature animals improved (~60%) in serum-free media but fewer than 10% of UE cells from immature rats attached. In no case did the UE cells proliferate at a rate equal to the rate of cell death and/or detachment. Effectively no cells remained attached by 96-120h.

It was demonstrated experimentally that an appropriate basement membrane-like substrate, i.e., Engelbreth Holm Swarm (EHS) tumor matrix, would significantly improve UE cell attachment (19). UE cell attachment at 24h was greater than 80%. Depending on their plating density immature UE cells proliferated to confluence within 48-72h after attachment (Fig. 3). However, the presence of this basement membrane matrix alone is not adequate to establish polarity. UE cells cultured on EHS matrix-covered wells detached after becoming confluent and were gone by days 12-14 (Fig. 3). Cells attaching at a density less than 250 cells/mm^2 experienced only two population doublings, and thus failed to become confluent (50). Since it had been demonstrated that, in addition to appropriate matrix relationships, important facets of epithelial cell function could be attributed to the availability of a permeable basal surface (29,49), UE cells were cultured on EHS matrix-impregnated Millicell HA filters (Millipore, Bedford, MA). UE cells cultured under these conditions in basal medium (2.5% FCS + 2.5% Nu-Serum) attached (>80%), proliferated to confluence and remained confluent for the course of the experiment (Fig. 3) (19).

The ability of primary UE cell cultures from immature (sexually naive) rats to establish and maintain polar organization was validated first by ultrastructural and immunocytochemical evidence. Transmission electron microscopy demonstrated that by the time UE cells cultured on EHS impregnated HA filters became confluent they were columnar, that junctional complexes including desmosomes were well developed between adjacent cells, and that cellular microvilli had elongated and become more numerous. Transepithelial resistance, >300 Ω/cm^2, had developed in post-confluent cells which had expressed <20 Ω/cm^2 in their preconfluent state (19). Polarized cells continued to express their signature profile of cytokeratins (#7,8,18,19). The effectiveness of the cell separation method was certified by the failure to detect any cytokeratin negative cells. The appearance of E-cadherin (uvomorulin) was restricted to the basolateral surface in post-confluent cells. *In vivo* appearance of E-cadherin, a plasma membrane protein associated exclusively with epithelial cells, is also limited to the basolateral plasma membrane (21). While the expression of E-cadherin restricted to the basolateral surface of the UE cell does indicate reorganization of the cell surface it cannot be used to prove complete separation of the plasma membrane domains of UE cells at this point.

In addition to these indices of morphological polarity there are indices of functional polarity which can be demonstrated in post-confluent UE cells (6,19). These are based on the same types of evidence used to establish polarization in established cell lines and include

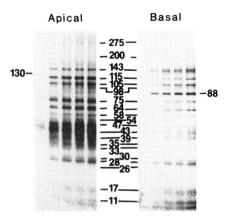

Figure 5. Apical and basal secretory profiles of UE cells cultured on EHS matrix covered filters for 11 days. Cells were labeled with [^{35}S]-methionine and apical and basal secretory compartments were harvested at 2,4,6,8 and 10h of incubation (left to right). Numbers designate the molecular mass (X10^{-3}) of the secretory products. Proteins common to both compartments are indicated in the center. Components that are either uniquely or preferentially secreted to a specific compartment are designated at the appropriate side. Secretion in both compartments was linear through 10 hours of incubation. The apical/basal ratio at each time point was 26 [From Glasser *et al* (19), with permission].

preferential uptake of amino acids (^{35}S-methionine) via the basal surface (Fig. 4A), and a significant increase in the total (apical + basal) secretory activity of the UE cell (Fig. 4B) which is primarily due to the increasing preference towards apical secretion (Fig. 4C) (45,46,49). Shortly after the cells become confluent the pH of the apical secretory chamber increases from 7.2 to 7.65 and that of the basal secretory chamber shifts from 7.2 to 7.09. This difference may reflect the establishment of a functional proton pump, and signifies the development of asymmetric distinctions between apical and basolateral surfaces.

The protein and glycoprotein profiles of the apical vs. basolateral secretory compartment which developed as a time-dependent function of polarity have been characterized by gel electrophoresis (Fig. 5). The fractional distribution of shared proteins and glycoproteins may vary between secretory compartments as a function of developmental polarity or in response to direct or paracrine regulatory signals. While the majority of proteins are distributed between both secretory compartments some proteins carry specific signals for unique or preferred polarized secretion. The significance of the preferential secretion of the 88Kd protein to the basal compartment (Fig. 5) lies not only in the protein itself (which remains to be characterized and assigned a role), for identification of this protein establishes that for the first time the profile of basal secretions of the UE cell can be described. It is now feasible to study putative signals transduced via the UE cell to the stroma. The first evidence for the preferential basal secretion of such a signal, i.e., PGF$_{2\alpha}$, has recently been obtained in this experimental cell system (Table 2; 22).

A notable characteristic of this polarized culture system which is a sequel of establishing morphological and functional polarity, is the apparent maintenance of hormonal responsiveness (19). Still to be determined is the extent to which the evolution of polarity and the degree of responsiveness to steroid hormones and other regulatory factors are related in UE and other epithelial cell systems. Data implicating changes in apical secretion in blastocyst development (43) and in basal secretions in transduction of deciduogenic signals (4,22) can be offered as proof of the correlation between hormonal regulation of UE cells and their phenotypic polarized expression. In valid culture systems this type of response should be evident in UE cells *in vitro*.

Table 2. $PGF_{2\alpha}$ and PGE Production by Polarized Uterine Epithelial Cells [from Jacobs et al. (22), with permission]

| | | ng/10^6 Cells[1] | | | |
| | | $PGF_{2\alpha}$[2] | | PGE | |
	Day of Confluence	Apical	Basal	Apical	Basal
Immature Mouse (2)	2	1.5 ± 0.3	3.8 ± 4.3	0.3 ± 0.0	0.5 ± 0.0
Immature Rat	4	1.1 ± 0.3	5.2 ± 3.0	0.1 ± 0.0	0.3 ± 0.0

[1]Net production over 4 hours, RIA.
[2]Cell associated $PGF_{2\alpha}$ is 5.4 ng ± .3 ng/10^6 cells

Specific secreted proteins and glycoproteins have been advanced as markers of estrogen action on the uterus (23,52,56). Uterine strips from hormone-treated immature rats secreted the 115 and 64 Kd subunits of the 180 Kd complement protein C_3 into the incubation medium (23,56). This same protein has been identified in the apical secretions of polarized UE cells cultured in complete medium on EHS covered HA filters (19). These data suggest that polarized cultures of UE cells, counter to their behavior in classic culture systems, not only respond to estrogen but do so in a manner similar to their response in vivo.

Despite the paucity of direct evidence it has generally been assumed that the transitional apical disposition of proteins and glycoproteins is not simply structural. Rather, changing patterns of morphological and biochemical components have been implicated in the shift of the UE cell from prereceptive to receptive. Nothing is really known about the blastocyst attachment reaction. Since both HS[PG] and those proteins that can specifically bind to adhesive molecules are components of the apical UE and trophectoderm surfaces it has been proposed, but not proven, that an interaction between the two cell types occurs at the adhesive stage of implantation (25). This type of binding interaction has been identified in other cell systems (11,24).

Studies of proteoglycan synthesis and secretion confirm the hormonal responsiveness of the polarized UE cell (6). Heparan sulfate containing proteoglycan (HS[PG]) and keratan sulfate proteoglycan (KSPG) are the main sulfated products secreted by the polarized UE cell (6). KSPG secretion paralleled the evolution of UE cell polarity; an increasing proportion of synthesized KSPG appears in the apical secretory compartment as a function of time. While most HS[PG] was secreted apically this was found to be independent of the development of polarity (Fig. 6). The patterns observed in polarized UE cells mimicked the secretory responses of estrogen stimulated uterine strips (9). It is of interest that the estrogen sensitivity of KSPG synthesis and secretion noted in isolated polarized UE cells could not be detected in the studies of whole uterine strips. Of the sulfated molecules secreted by UE cells, 80-90% are directed to the apical surface. Preferential apical secretion is consonant with other studies which show HS[PG] expression at the luminal surface of mouse uteri (31,53). Information concerning vectorial secretion of glycoconjugates by polarized cells has primarily been obtained through the study of viral glycoproteins in infected cell lines (28). There is only minimal data concerning the production and vectorial movement of proteins and glycoproteins of host epithelia which would be more applicable to the study of UE cell receptivity. Even fewer studies have focused on the subject of basal secretion although secreted HS[PG] can be integrated both structurally and functionally into the basal lamina whose composition can also be altered by basal secretion (5). In the absence of an appropriate experimental cell system none of this provocative information could be applied to the definition of the regulatory biology of the receptive UE cell and its role in the transduction of deciduogenic stimuli. The short transitional length of the receptive period has been attributed to the estrogen stimulated turnover of UE cell assoc-

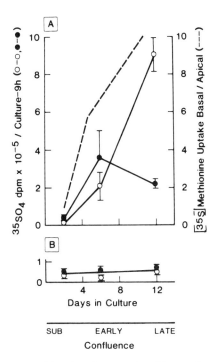

Figure 6. Sulfated glycoconjugates secreted by subconfluent, early and late confluent cultures of uterine epithelial cells. Cell density, measured in parallel cultures, ranged from 2500-3000 cells/mm^2, from culture day 2 through 13. Secreted radiolabeled glycoconjugates (H$_2$[^{35}S]O$_4$, 9 hours) were analyzed as described by Carson *et al.* (6). Secretory patterns of keratan sulfate proteoglycan (○) and heparan sulfate bearing molecules (●) are shown for both the apical (A) and basal (B) plasma membrane secretory compartments. The dashed line represents the ratio of ^{35}S-methionine uptake from the basal vs. the apical surface of similar cultures over this same time period (see Fig. 4A; 19).

iated proteoglycans (31,53). If attachment fails to occur the receptive phase is sequentially transposed to a refractory period. The occurrence of this second non-receptive phase represents a further shift in the composition of the UE cell (32; Fig. 2) implying a related change in the apical plasma membrane of the UE cell which will not support blastocyst attachment.

No satisfactory model for *in vitro* implantation exists. None of the temporal or hormonal constraints which regulate blastocyst attachment *in utero* appear to influence blastocysts *in vitro* (13,16,39). As long as blastocysts *in vitro* are provided with optimal nutritive conditions for at least 24h they will become adhesive, attach without discrimination to almost any surface (explants of whole uteri or endometrium, to cultures of endometrial cells, to coatings of collagen I, fibronectin, laminin or even to bare tissue culture plastic), and undergo trophoblast outgrowth (48). This autonomous *in vitro* behavior has been attributed to the failure of classical culture systems to maintain the three-dimensional architecture found *in utero* (10,47). Cell culture models which restore UE cell polarity provide the basis for hormonal regulation and expression of the specific functions of UE cells. These systems could serve as relevant experimental models for *in vitro* implantation.

In Vitro **Non-receptivity and Estrogen**

In pilot experiments to assess the utility of polarized UE cell cultures as models for *in vitro* implantation, blastocysts recovered from the uteri of pregnant rats on the day of

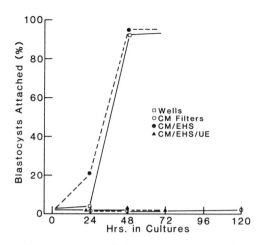

Figure 7. *In vitro* attachment of rat blastocysts to adhesive and non-adhesive surfaces. Blastocysts recovered from the uteri of pregnant rats on the day of implantation were transferred to various culture surfaces. *In vitro* culture was under conditions optimally favorable to attachment in complete medium (19) with only estradiol-17β at physiological concentrations. After 48 hours in culture >90% of the blastocysts attached to bare plastic wells (□) but none attached to bare CM filters (○). In more than 95% of the cases attachment was followed by trophoblast outgrowth. If CM filters were initially covered with EHS matrix (●) 92% of the transferred blastocysts attached and underwent trophoblast outgrowth. However, if a polarized uterine epithelial cell culture was first established on EHS covered CM filters before blastocysts were transferred no embryos attached under these culture conditions (▲).

implantation were transferred to different culture surfaces (Fig. 7) and cultured in completemedium (19). Estrogen is present in physiological concentrations in this medium which contains 2.5% FCS and 2.5% Nu-Serum. All other steroids are below their physiological range. After 48h in culture 90% of the blastocysts attached to bare plastic wells; trophoblast outgrowth followed in over 95% of the attached embryos. Not a single blastocyst attached to the bare CM filter. However, if the CM filter was first covered with EHS matrix (CM/EHS) 92% of the blastocysts attached and underwent trophoblast outgrowth. To test the ability of the blastocysts to attach, embryos were transferred to other culture surfaces either 48 or 72h after culture on bare CM filters (Figs. 7,8). Within 24h of transfer to EHS matrix covered CM filters more than 80% of the embryos had attached (Fig 8, CM/EHS). Of critical importance to this study was the behavior of embryos cultured with UE cells polarized on EHS covered CM filters (CM/EHS/UE). None of the embryos attached to polarized UE cells over the course of the experiment (Fig. 8, CM/EHS/UE).

Blastocysts which failed to attach to polarized UE cells cultured on EHS covered CM filters (CM/EHS/UE, Figs. 7,8,9) may have been impaired in some manner. However, when the same embryos were removed after 48h on polarized epithelial cells (CM/EHS/UE) and transferred to CM filters covered only with EHS matrix (CM/EHS) more than 80% attached within 24h (Fig. 9). Additional groups of unattached blastocysts were transferred after 24, 48 or 72h from polarized UE cell cultures (CM/EHS/UE) to EHS covered CM filters on which uterine stromal (US) cells rather than UE cells comprised the monolayer (CM/EHS/US). At least 95% of the transferred embryos attached to the stromal cells (Fig. 9). The experiments proved that the embryos were always competent and retained their ability to attach.

These preliminary data validate this experimental cell model as a reasonably faithful model for *in vitro* implantation. The responsiveness of polarized UE cells has allowed, for the first time, the imposition of constraints on the *in vitro* attachment of viable adhesive blastocysts. The presence of estrogen appears to render the UE cell, but not the US cell, non-receptive to blastocyst attachment.

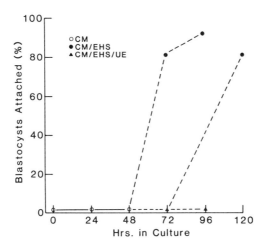

Figure 8. Transfer of blastocysts from bare CM filters. To determine if blastocysts originally cultured on bare CM filters (○) retained their competence to attach they were transferred, after 48h, to CM filters covered with EHS matrix (●). Over 80% of the blastocysts attached during the next 24 hours. Another group of embryos was transferred to polarized uterine epithelial cells in matrix covered filters (▲). None attached but 80% of a subgroup retransferred to matrix covered CM filters (no cells) attached during the next 24-30 hours. Culture conditions were identical to Fig 6.

In spite of certain constitutive limitations the analyses of *in vitro* cultures of separated endometrial cell types has yielded new data and provided insights regarding the regulatory biology of the uterus, particularly the expression of specialized functions by epithelial and stromal cells. The utility of these polarized cultures of primary, unpassaged cells is enhanced by experimental and analytical access to both the apical and basolateral surface domains of the epithelial cell. This experimental cell system provides advantages not afforded by the use of conventional *in vitro* and *in vivo* methods. Polarized UE cells apparently respond to steroid hormones and differentiate *in vitro*. Direct response, vis-a-vis indirect instructive or permissive stromal signals, is a major element of hormone action in cultured UE cells from post-neonatal rats. Hormonally responsive differentiation is demonstrated by changing protein and glycoprotein profiles of the apical and basal UE secretory compartments which include secretion of putative estrogen markers (23,26,56). These data modify the concept, derived from studies of long-term fetal or neonatal epithelial tissue-stromal tissue recombinations, which states that epithelial cell differentiation is a product of indirect hormone action mediated by stromal cells (8).

Coupling these responsive uterine epithelial cells (6,19) with uterine stromal cells cultured *in vitro* (17,18) it will now be possible to construct cell-cell recombinations rather than tissue-tissue recombinations. Cell-cell recombinations offer the advantage of being morphologically and functionally responsive over short periods of time. Epithelial cell-stromal cell recombinations (homotypic, heterotypic, synchronous, asynchronous) can be used to evaluate the relative importance of epithelial to stromal as well as stromal to epithelial paracrine intercommunication. Thus, it will be possible to place the role of epithelial to stromal communication in cell-substratum interactions and in the transduction of signals to initiate the differentiation of the stromal cell in perspective (20). This framework allows the definition not only of the influence of steroid hormones but of other regulatory factors (growth factors, cytokines, lymphokines, antigen presenting cells) on the evolution of uterine receptivity and the subsequent, interdependent processes by which pregnancy is established in the mammal.

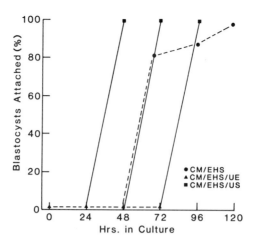

Figure 9. Blastocysts which fail to attach to polarized uterine epithelial cells (▼) remain competent to attach. When these blastocysts are transferred after 24,48 or 72 hours to uterine stromal monolayers on EHS matrix impregnated filters in the same culture environment (Figs. 6,7) nearly all attach within 24 hours (■). Unattached blastocysts transferred from polarized uterine epithelial cells to matrix covered CM filters also attach successfully (●).

Acknowledgements

The authors thank Dr. Shaila Mani and Dr. Fernand Leroy for their thoughtful discussions of this work. Mrs. Carolyn Armijo (wordprocessing), Mrs. Debbie Townley (photography) and Mr. David Scarff (illustration) made contributions that are most appreciated. This research was supported by grants from the National Institutes of Health to S.R. Glasser (HD-22785, HD-25189) and to the Center for Population Research and Reproductive Biology (HD-07495). J. Mulholland was supported by a grant from the Lalor Foundation.

References

1. Anderson, T.L., Olson, G.E. and Hoffman, L.H., Stage-specific alterations in the apical membrane glycoproteins of endometrial epithelial cells related to implantation. Biol. Reprod. 34:701 (1986).

2. Betteridge, K.J., Embryo Transfer in Farm Animals. A Review of Techniques and Applications. Agriculture Canada Monograph 16 (1977).

3. Bissell, M.J., Hall, H.C. and Parry, G., How does the extracellular matrix direct gene expression? J. Theor. Biol. 99:31 (1982).

4. Cao, Z.-B., Jones, M.A. and Harper, M.J.K., Prostaglandin translocation from the lumen of the rabbit uterus *in vitro* in relation to the day of pregnancy or pseudopregnancy. Biol. Reprod. 31:505 (1984).

5. Caplan, M.J., Stow, J.L., Newman, A.P., Madri, J., Anderson, H.C., Farquhar, M.G., Palade, G.E. and Jameson, J., Dependence on pH of polarized sorting of secreted proteins. Nature (Lond.) 329:623 (1987).

6. Carson, D.D., Tang., J.-Y., Julian, J.A. and Glasser, S.R., Vectorial secretion of proteoglycans by polarized rat uterine epithelial cells. J. Cell Biol. 107:2425 (1988).

7. Chang, M.C., Development and fate of transferred rabbit ova or blastocysts in relation to ovulation time of recipients. J. Exp. Zool. 14:197 (1950).

8. Cunha, G.R., Chung, L.W.K., Shannon, J.M., Taguchi, O. and Fujii, H., Hormone induced morphogenesis and growth: role of mesenchymal-epithelial interactions. Rec. Prog. Horm. Res. 39:559 (1983).

9. Dutt, A.J., Tang, J.-P., Welply, J.K. and Carson, D.D., Regulation of N-linked glycoprotein assembly in uteri by steroid hormones. Endocrinology 118:661 (1986).

10. Enders, A.C., Chavez, D.J. and Schlafke, S., Comparisons of implantation *in utero* and *in vitro*. In: Cellular and Molecular Aspects of Implantation. S.R. Glasser and D.W. Bullock, eds., Plenum Press, New York (1981), p. 365.

11. Farach, M.C., Tang, J.-P., Decker, G.L. and Carson, D.D., Heparin/heparan sulfate is involved in attachment and spreading of mouse embryos *in vitro*. Dev. Biol. 123:401 (1987).

12. Glasser, S.R., Biochemical and structural changes in uterine endometrial cell types following natural or artificial deciduogenic stimuli. Troph. Res. 4 (1989), in press.

13. Glasser, S.R. and Clark, J.H.. A determinant role for progesterone in the development of uterine sensitivity to decidualization and ovoimplantation. In: Developmental Biology of Reproduction. C.L. Markert and J. Papaconstantinou, eds., Academic Press, New York (1975), p. 311.

14. Glasser, S.R. and McCormack, S.A., Estrogen-modulated uterine gene transcription in relation to decidualization. Endocrinology 104:1112 (1979).

15. Glasser, S.R. and McCormack, S.A., Functional development of rat trophoblast and decidual cells during establishment of the hemochorial placenta. Adv. Biosciences 25:165 (1979).

16. Glasser, S.R. and McCormack, S.A., Cellular and molecular aspects of decidualization and implantation. In: Proteins and Steroids in Early Pregnancy. H.M. Beier and P. Karlson, eds., Springer-Verlag, Berlin (1982), p. 245.

17. Glasser, S.R. and Julian, J.A., Intermediate filament protein as a marker for uterine stromal cell decidualization. Biol. Reprod. 35:463 (1986).

18. Glasser, S.R., Lampelo, S., Munir, M.I. and Julian, J.A., Expression of desmin, laminin and fibronectin during *in situ* differentiation (decidualization) of rat uterine stromal cells. Differentiation 35:132 (1987).

19. Glasser, S.R., Julian, J.A., Decker, G.L., Tang, J.-Y. and Carson, D.D., Development of morphological and functional polarity in primary cultures of immature rat uterine epithelial cells. J. Cell Biol. 107:2409 (1988).

20. Glasser, S.R., Julian, J.A., Mani, S.K., Mulholland, J., Munir, M.I., Lampelo, S. and Soares, M.J., Blastocyst-endometrial relationships: reciprocal int the maintenance of oestradiol-induced inhibition of uterine sensitivity in the ovariectomized rat. J. Endocrinol. 46:341 (1970).

31. Morris, J.E., Potter, S.W. and Gaza-Bulesco, G., Estradiol induces an accumulation of free heparan sulfate glycosaminoglycan chains in uterine epithelium. Endocrinology 122:242 (1988).

32. Mulholland, J. and Leroy, F., Protein and mRNA synthesis in the peri-implantation rat endometrium. In: Blastocyst Implantation. K. Yoshinaga, ed., Adams Publishing Group, Boston (1989), p. 31.

33. McCormack, S.A. and Glasser, S.R., Differential response of individual uterine cell types from immature rats treated with estradiol. Endocrinology 106:1634 (1980).

34. McLaren, A. and Michie, D., Studies on the transfer of fertilized mouse eggs to foster mothers. I. Factors affecting the implantation and survival of native and transferred eggs. J. Exp. Biol. 33:394-416 (1956).

35. Newcomb, R. and Rowson, L.E.A., Conception rate after transfer of cow eggs in relation to synchronization of oestrus and age of egg. J. Reprod. Fertil. 43:539 (1975).

36. Noyes, R.W., Dickmann, Z. and Gates, A.H., Ovum transfers, synchronous and asynchronous, in the study of implantation. In: Delayed Implantation. A.C. Enders, ed., Univ. of Chicago Press, Chicago (1963), p. 197.

37. Polge, C., Embryo transplantation and preservation. In: Control of Pig Reproduction. D.J.A. Cole and G.R. Foxworth, eds., Butterworth Scientific, London (1982), p. 277.

38. Pope, W.F., Uterine synchrony: a cause of embryonic loss. Biol. Reprod. 39:999 (1988).

39. Psychoyos, A., Endocrine control of egg implantation. In: Handbook of Physiology, Sect. 7. Endocrinology Vol. II, Pt. II, R.O. Greep and E.B. Astwood, eds. Am. Physiol. Soc., Washington, D.C. (1973), p.187.

40. Psychoyos, A., Hormonal control of ovoimplantation. Vitam. Horm. 32:201 (1974).

41. Psychoyos, A., Uterine receptivity for nidation. Ann. N.Y., Acad. Sci. 476:36 (1986).

42. Rapraeger, A., Jalkansen, M. and Bernfield, M., Cell surface proteoglycan associates with the cytoskeleton at the basolateral cell surface in mouse mammary epithelial cells. J. Cell Biol. 103:2683 (1986).

43. Roberts, R.M. and Bazer, F.W., The functions of uterine secretions. J. Reprod. Fertil. 82:875 (1988).

44. Roberts, R.M., Schalue-Francis, T., Francis, H. and Keisler, D., Maternal recognition of pregnancy and embryonic loss. Theriogenol. 33:175 (1990).

45. Rodriquez-Boulan, E. and Nelson, W.J., Morphogenesis of the polarized epithelial cell phenotype. Science 245:718 (1989).

46. Sabatini, D.D., Griepp, E.B., Boulan-Rodriguez, E., Dolan, J.J., Robbins, S., Papadopolous, S., Ivanov, I.E. and Rindler, M.J., Biogenesis of epithelial cell polarity. Mod. Cell Biol. 2:419 (1983).

47. Sengupta, J., Given, R.L., Carey, J.B., Weitlauf, H.M., Primary culture of mouse endometrium on floating collagen gels: a potential *in vitro* model for implantation. Ann. N.Y. Acad. Sci. 476:75 (1986).

48. Sherman, M.I. and Matthaei, K.I., Factors involved in implantation-related events *in vitro*. Prog. Reprod. Biol. 7:43 (1980).

49. Simons, K. and Fuller, S.D., Cell surface polarity in epithelia. Annu. Rev. Cell Biol. 1:243 (1985).

50. Smith, J.A. and Martin, L., Regulation of cell proliferation. In: Cell Cycle Controls. G.M. Padella, I.L. Cameron and A. Zimmerman, eds., Academic Press (1974), p. 43.

51. Tachi, C., Tachi, S. and Lindner, H.R., Modification by progesterone of oestradiol-induced cell proliferation, RNA synthesis and oestradiol distribution in the uterus. J. Reprod. Fertil. 31:59 (1972).

52. Takeda, A., Takahashi, N. and Shimazu, S., Identification and characterization of an estrogen-inducible glycoprotein (USP-1) synthesized and secreted by rat uterine epithelial cells. Endocrinology 122:105 (1988).

53. Tang, J.-Y., Julian, J., Glasser, S.R. and Carson, D.D., Heparan sulphate proteoglycan synthesis and metabolism by mouse uterine epithelial cells cultured *in vitro*. J. Biol. Chem. 262:12832 (1987).

54. Watson, J., Anderson, F.B., Alam, E., O'Grady, J.E. and Heald, P.J., Plasma hormones and pituitary luteinizing hormone in the rat during the early stages of pregnancy and after post-coital treatment with tamoxifen (ICI 46,474). J. Endocrinol. 65:7 (1975).

55. Webel, S.K., Peters, J.B. and Anderson, L.L., Synchronous and asynchronous transfer of embryos in the pig. J. Anim. Sci. 30:565 (1970).

56. Wheeler, C., Komm, B.S. and Lyttle, C.R., Estrogen regulation of protein synthesis in the immature rat uterus: the effects of progesterone during *in vitro* incubation. Endocrinology 120:910 (1987).

Questions

Dr. Stancel: Have you done anything with calcium modulators, or similar substances?

Dr. Glasser: No we haven't, largely because until NIH smiled upon us just this winter, we didn't have the money to do it. We have used the rabbit, though, and progesterone induces an increase in the incorporation of label and estrogen has no obvious effect on control values. The total secretion goes down but the basal secretion increases ten-fold. Is it a viable system? Out the apical side comes all the uteroglobin that Joe Daniel would ever want to see in his life. So it is a viable system, and the most exciting thing is that in the superficial implanter it has a different strategy. The cell, responding to the same hormones, does different things on either side. Now I can also tell you that when we do a dose-response curve that the basal side is an order of magnitude more sensitive to each of the hormones than is the apical side. So you'll get a change in the rat on the basal side using estrogen at 1×10^{-11}, and it takes 1×10^{-10} on the apical side. We get new data each day that makes us scratch our head and wonder which way to go with this. But right now, given its limitations, it's one of the more exciting models that we have. We're getting ready to do *in vitro* implantation using the rabbit model.

Dr. Larson: Dr. Glasser, you have shown the effect of estrogen, but what about the effect of estrogen on nidation?

Dr. Glasser: What we're doing now is trying to mimic estrous estrogen, not nidatory estrogen. We haven't yet done those experiments in a way that we're comfortable with, in a way that we can mimic nidatory estrogen. The problem is to get specific attachment. If we got attachment with estrogen and no attachment with progesterone we'd have to do several control studies to insure we were getting specific attachment. One of the ways we seek to do this is to identify the protein or glycoprotein that is stage-specific, then we hope to make a monoclonal, perhaps a monospecific antibody and set up some sort of blocking assay. If we could get up to 85% inhibition at the right time, under the right conditions on the right cell side, then we could talk about true biological effects rather than nonspecific adhesion, which is a big pothole to fall into.

Dr. Leavitt: Stan, concerning your progesterone treatment, have you tried this with progesterone alone for a long enough period to see if you could get a progesterone specific set of proteins?

Dr. Glasser: Well, let's put it this way. We've done one-dimensional gels and inspected them. We are now doing computerized densitometric analysis. And the data that is beginning to come out suggests that for each of the hormones there is a specific profile. But we have not compared the results using estrogen and progesterone alone versus the combination of the two hormones.

Dr. Carson: This isn't really a question, I just wanted to clarify the indomethacin data. What goes on with indomethacin in uterine epithelial cells that are polarized is that you have substantial intracellular pools of prostaglandin f2-α and that is not the case with the nonpolarized cells.

8

Uterine Extracellular Matrix Remodeling in Pregnancy

I. Damjanov[1] and U.M. Wewer[2]
Department of Pathology and Cell Biology
Thomas Jefferson University, Philadelphia, Pennsylvania 19107[1]
The University Institute of Pathological Anatomy, Copenhagen, Denmark[2]

Summary

As an early response to hormones of pregnancy the uterine stroma undergoes a complex set of changes known as decidual reaction, leading to the formation of a nodular deciduoma in rodents or a decidual membrane in humans. Decidualization leads to striking changes in the size and shape of stromal uterine cells, accompanied by changes in their function and synthetic profile. The decidual cells synthesize and deposit in the extracellular spaces laminin, collagen type IV, heparan sulfate proteoglycan and entactin which are assembled into morphologically distinct pericellular basement membranes. It is proposed that the pericellular basement membranes in the decidua serve multiple functions and among others mediate the implantation of the embryo, provide the substrate for the early embryogenesis and at the same time form a membrane delimiting the embryo from the maternal organism.

Introduction

The endometrial stromal cells of the eutherian uterus respond to hormones of pregnancy and undergo a set of complex changes collectively known as decidualization (1). In humans, decidual cells form a membrane, whereas in rodents the proliferating hormonally primed stroma forms a tumor-like nodule called deciduoma (13).

The function of decidual cells has not been fully elucidated, and it is thought that they play a role in regulating the implantation, the invasion of trophoblast; the establishment of and subsequent maintenance of the uteroplacental unit; and the protection of the embryo from the maternal immune system (1,3,7). During the decidualization the stromal cells enlarge and rearrange their cytoskeleton (4,11) begin secreting hormones (10) and various other proteins whose function has not yet been fully elucidated (2,5,9). The extracellular matrix also changes in this process, becomes more abundant and qualitatively different from the matrix surrounding the stromal cells of the nonpregnant uterus (3,8,10). The biological significance of these changes is mostly unknown, although judging from their magnitude one could assume that the stromal changes are important for the initiation and maintenance of the intrauterine stages of pregnancy.

In this contribution we are focusing on: 1. the sequential changes leading to the formation of the decidua in humans; 2. pericellular basement membrane formation in the murine deciduoma; and 3. comparison between human and murine decidual response.

Decidualization of the Human Endometrial Stroma

Mature human decidua of early as well as late pregnancy is composed of large decidual cells and prominent extracellular matrix arranged into basement membrane (BM) like

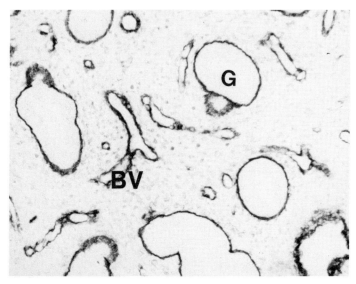

Figure 1.   Human endometrium in the proliferative phase of the menstrual cycle reacted with antibodies to laminin. Linear staining is seen outlining the glands (G). Blood vessels (BV) are also delimited with a laminin-rich basement membrane. The stromal cells are unreactive. Immunoperoxidase technique. x 160.

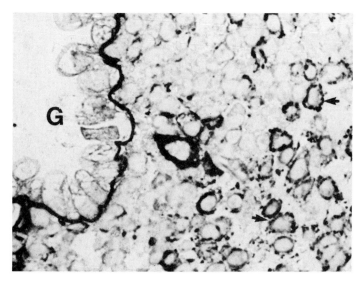

Figure 2. Human decidua from early stages of pregnancy reacted with antibodies to laminin. In addition to the linear staining of the epithelial basement membrane delimiting the gland (G), immunoreactivity is seen along the cell membrane of individual intermediate size decidual cells (arrows). Immunoperoxidase technique. x 240.

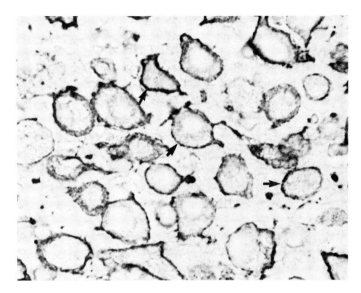

Figure 3. Large mature decidual cells from early stages of pregnancy reacted with antibodies to laminin. Circumferential reactivity is seen along individual large decidual cells (arrows). Indirect immunoperoxidase technique. x 280.

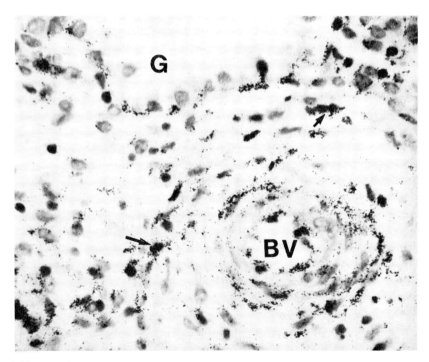

Figure 4. Human early pregnancy decidua exposed to in situ hybridization with a radioactive cDNA probe to B-1 laminin chain. Radioactivity, indicative of specific RNA is seen in epithelial cells of the gland (G), vascular cells (BV) and scattered decidual cells (arrows). In situ hybridization autoradiography. x 240.

pericellular sheaths (3). Like the basement membranes in other sites the matrix of mature decidua contains the typical collagenous and non-collagenous macromolecules: collagen type IV, laminin, heparan sulfate proteoglycan, entactin, and fibronectin (8,14).

The formation of the pericellular BM is a continuous process that intensifies gradually during the nine months of pregnancy. In the nonpregnant uterus the stromal cells resemble the fibroblasts phenotypically and the extracellular spaces contain banded collagen fibrils rather than matrix assembled into basement membranes. In the stroma of the nonpregnant uterine endometrium there is no immunohistochemically demonstrable collagen type IV or laminin, except in the perivascular spaces and at the interface between the stroma and the glandular epithelium. The formation of pericellular membranes appears to be coincidental with changes in stromal cell morphology. As the pregnancy advances the stromal cells gradually enlarge and shortly after implantation one can already discern three groups of decidual cells: large mature polygonal cells measuring more than 25 μm in diameter; medium-sized polygonal or round decidual cells measuring 15-25 μm in diameter, preferentially located close by the dilated and contorted endometrial glands; and small elongated cells measuring less than 15 μm in diameter resembling the fibroblasts or stromal cells from nonpregnant uteri. It was hypothesized that the medium-sized and large decidual cells evolve from the small elongated cells (14), as suggested by the fact that with advancing duration of the pregnancy there were more of large and fewer of small elongated cells. After the sixth week and to the end of the pregnancy the decidua consists predominately of large mature cells, the ratio for the large, intermediate and small cells being 10:3:0.1.

Immunohistochemical studies of nonpregnant endometrium disclosed collagen type IV, laminin, heparan sulfate proteoglycan and fibronectin colocalized in the basement membranes of the uterine glands and blood vessels (Figure 1). Stromal cells do not contain, nor are they surrounded by, these basement membrane components. Occasionally some minor pericellular aggregates of laminin could be seen in the late secretory predecidual endometrium. In the pregnant uteri, glands remain surrounded by the BM separating them from stromal cells that are unreactive with antibodies to either of the major components. However, along the cell membrane of the intermediate sized decidual cells there are granular deposits of laminin, type IV collagen, heparan sulfate, proteoglycan and fibronectin (Figure 2), which focally appear confluent encasing these cells. Ultrastructurally, the intermediate sized cells appear to be surrounded by a thin pericellular coat indistinguishable from the typical lamina densa of BM. Occasional larger 200-500 nm clumps of similar material are also seen between the cells. Although we do not have ultrastructural immunocytochemical data to definitively prove that the pericellular material is the product of the intermediate sized decidual cells, these cells show ultrastructural evidence of secretory activity and the close apposition of the pericellular matrix is most consistent with the view that it has been produced by these cells.

Large mature decidual cells are spaced at a distance from one another and are characteristically surrounded individually with a continuous BM that contains laminin, collagen type IV, fibronectin and heparan sulfate proteoglycan. These substances form a continuous pericellular basement membrane completely encircling each decidual cell (Figure 3). Ultrastructurally the pericellular matrix is arranged in a typical BM, that has a laminina rara and a lamina densa. Thus, one may conclude that the decidual cells not only secrete the typical basement membrane components, but that they assemble them into a morphologically distinct pericellular structure indistinguishable from BM in other locations.

Short term cultures of human decidua from early pregnancy revealed active synthesis of all major BM components (16). These data were corroborated by in situ hybridization, in which we have used a radioactive cDNA probe to human laminin B-1 chain to evaluate the synthetic activity of various cells in the pregnant uteri. As shown autoradiographically in Fig. 4, specific RNA indicative of B-1 chain laminin synthesis could be demonstrated in the glandular epithelium, blood vessel wall and in the scattered decidualized stromal cells. It appears that this secretory activity is hormonally regulated as suggested by immunohistochemical studies.

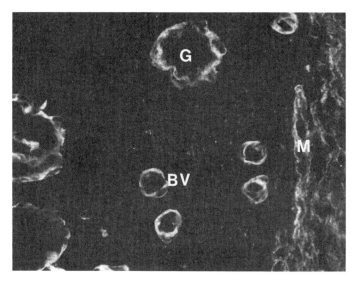

Figure 5.   Nonpregnant mouse uterus reacted with antibody to laminin. Laminin is seen in the basement membrane of the glands (G), vessel (BV) and the smooth muscle of the myometrium (M). Endometrial stromal cells are unreactive. Indirect immunofluorescene technique. x 160.

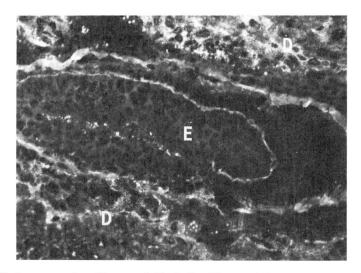

Figure 6.   Six day mouse embryo (E) surrounded by decidua (D), reacted with the antibody to heparan sulfate proteoglycan. In addition to embryonic basement membranes, immunoreactivity is seen in the decidua as well. Indirect immunofluorescence technique. x 240.

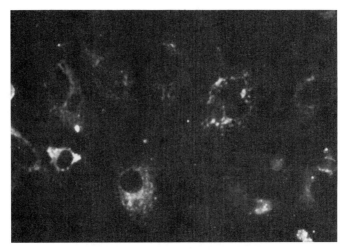

Figure 7.   Nonpregnant mouse endometrial cells explanted *in vitro* and reacted with the antibody to laminin two days after plating. Granular intracytoplasmic reactivity is seen in some cells indicating that the cells synthesize laminin. Indirect immunofluorescence technique. x 320.

Decidual cells explanted *in vitro* synthesize BM components in a manner that is comparable to the production *in vivo* (8,10). Like the matrix formed *in vivo*, laminin deposited between the explanted cells may serve as an anchoring material.   If the trophoblastic cells are cultured with decidual cells, they attach to the extracellular matrix suggesting that laminin or some other component of this matrix mediates attachment of the trophoblastic cells regulating the implantation and the depth of invasion (10).   The details of the interaction between laminin and the trophoblastic cells are not known.

Extracellular Matrix in Murine Decidua

In response to hormones of pregnancy and the signals transmitted by the embryos that have entered the uterine cavity, the stromal cells in the endometrium of rodents undergo proliferation and form a defined circumscribed nodule known as deciduoma (13). Similar nodules can be induced mechanically in hormonally primed uteri.   Stromal cells can spontaneously differentiate into decidual cells upon explantation*in vitro* (1).

In the non-pregnant uterus BM surround glands, vessels and individual smooth muscle cells of the myometrium (Figure 5). Normal non-pregnant uterine stromal cells resemble fibroblasts and do not produce immunohistochemically detectable laminin or collagen type IV. Instead, stroma contains collagen type I, III and VI (6). The onset of deciduoma formation is hall-marked by deposition of extracellular matrix rich on laminin, collagen type IV, fibronectin, heparan sulfate proteoglycan (Figure 6) and entactin (12,13). The basement membrane components are synthesized and deposited in the extracellular spaces by the decidualized stromal cells, indicating that these cells have not only changed their morphology but the synthetic profile as well.

Isolated stromal cells explanted *in vitro* undergo spontaneously decidual reaction and concomitantly with this transformation (13) begin secreting laminin and collagen type IV (Figure 7). This indicates that decidualization stimulates endometrial stromal cells to change their phenotype and also activate a new set of genes. Murine decidualization is in this respect similar to pregnancy related changes in the human endometrium (12,13).

Conclusion

Decidual cells of man and mouse actively synthesize basement membrane components such as laminin, fibronectin, collagen type IV entactin and heparan sulfate proteoglycan. The onset of basement membrane component production coincides with implantation. The newly synthesized basement membranes are deposited around individual decidual cells. It is suggested that this extracellular matrix mediates intercellular adhesion of decidual cells and at the same time facilitates the implantation of the embryo and regulates the extent of invasion of the trophoblast into the uterus.

References

1. Bell, S.C., Decidualization: regional differentiation and associated function. Oxford Rev. Reprod. Biol., 5:220 (1983).
2. Bell, S.C., Decidualization and insulin-like growth factor IGF binding protein: implications for its role in stromal cell differentiation and the decidual cell in haemochorial placentation. Hum. Reprod., 4:125 (1989).
3. Damjanov, I., Editorial: Vesalius and Hunter were right: decidua is a membrane. Lab. Invest., 53:597 (1985).
4. Glasser, S.R. and Julian, J., Intermediate filament protein as a marker of uterine stromal cell decidualization. Biol. Reprod. 35:463 (1986).
5. Jayatilak, P.G., Puryear, T.K., Herz, Z., Fazleabas, A., and Gibori, G., Protein secretion by mesometrial and antimesometrial rat decidual tissue: evidence for differential gene expression. Endocrinology 125:659 (1989).
6. Karkavelas, G., Kefalides, N.A., Amenta, P.S., and Martinez-Hernandez, A., Comparative ultrastructural localization of collagen types III, IV, VI and laminin in rat uterus and kidney. J. Ultrastruct. Mol. Struct. Res. 100:137 (1988).
7. Kearns, M. and Lala, P.K., Life history of decidual cells: a review. Am. J. Reprod. Immunol. 3:78 (1983).
8. Kisalus, L., Herr, J.C., and Little, C.D., Immunolocalization of extracellular matrix proteins and collagen synthesis in first-trimester human decidua. Anat. Rec., 218:402 (1987).
9. Leavitt, W.W., MacDonald, R.G., and Shwaery, G.T., Characterization of deciduoma marker proteins in hamster uterus: detection in decidual cell cultures. Biol. Reprod. 2:631 (1985).
10. Loke, Y.W., Gardner, L., Burland, K., and King, A., Laminin in human trophoblast-decidua interaction. Hum. Reprod., 4:457 (1989).
11. Ridick, D.H., Daly, D.C., and Walters, C.A., The uterus as an endocrine compartment. Clinics Perinatol., 10:627 (1983).
12. von Koskull, H. and Virtanen, I., Induction of cytokeratin expression in human mesenchymal cells. J. Cell. Physiol. 133:321 (1987).
13. Wan, Y-J., Wu, T-C., Chung, A.E., and Damjanov, I., Monoclonal antibodies to laminin reveal the heterogeneity of basement membranes in the developing and adult mouse tissues. J. Cell. Biol. 98:971 (1984).
14. Welsh, A.O. and Enders, A.C., Light and electron microscopic examination of the mature decidual cells of the rat with emphasis on the antimesometrial decidua and its degeneration. Am. J. Anat. 172:1 (1985).
15. Wewer, U.M., Damjanov, A., Weiss, J., Liotta, L.A., and Damjanov, I., Mouse endometrial stromal cells produce basement-membrane components. Differentiation 32:39 (1986).
16. Wewer, U.M., Faber, M., Liotta, L.A., and Albrechtsen, R., Immunochemical and ultrastructural assessment of the nature of the pericellular basement of human decidual cells. Lab. Invest. 53:624 (1985).

Questions

Dr. Glasser: I would ask you whether substances like laminin act as separators, barriers or facilitators of stromal-epithelial cell interactions?

Dr. Damjanov: Dan Carson has good experimental evidence that laminin is a sticky molecule. There are actually circulating cells in the mouse which express laminin. We know of at least three major laminin binding proteins which are expressed on the surface of tumor cells, and we have cloned one of these "receptors" and have shown that it is also expressed in the embryo. This sticking, of course, is a two way street, and I think that this sticking must also send a message into the blastocyst itself and turns on a whole sort of metabolic changes that might assist in penetration or are some other event. This is really a complex issue.

Dr. Carson: I think you have pretty impressive evidence that the components of the extracellular matrix markedly influences how a cell behaves. Have you done any experiments using antibodies specific for particular laminin chains, like B-1 versus B-2 chains to see if the relative composition of those chains change in the uterus during implantation.

Dr. Damjanov: No we haven't, but I need to elaborate on this question. The three chains of laminin are not synthesized coincidentally. So during, for example, embryonic development, the B chain is the first to appear and then the A chain appears. So one could assume that in a rapidly developing system like the decidua, there is a discordant expression of these chains.

9

Glycoprotein Expression and Function in Embryo-Uterine Interactions

D. D. Carson, N. Raboudi and A. L. Jacobs
Department of Biochemistry and Molecular Biology
The University of Texas M. D. Anderson Cancer Center
Houston, Texas   77030

Summary

The interactions that occur among embryonic and uterine cells during the implantation process are dramatic examples of highly-regulated cell adhesion events.   Evidence has accumulated over the past few years implicating the involvement of glycoproteins of both embryonic and uterine cell surfaces in these interactions.   Notably, heparan sulfate proteoglycans (HSPG), integrins, lactosaminoglycans and their receptors as well as a variety of other components of the extracellular matrix have the capacity to support aspects of cell adhesion in this system. From the standpoint of the embryo, glycoprotein expression appears to be regulated by the developmental clock of the embryo, such that HSPG- and integrin-dependent cell adhesion systems are expressed early relative to certain other cell adhesion systems.   In the uterus, there appear to be a number of factors that influence patterns of glycoprotein expression. These include steroid hormones, maturational factors and potential embryonic influences.   Uterine epithelial cells are even more complex with regard to regulation of glycoprotein expression.   In addition to the considerations described above, the apical and basolateral cell surface domains of uterine epithelial cells exhibit a marked difference in their respective patterns of glycoprotein expression.   Furthermore, different glycoproteins are metabolized at different rates and by different pathways within these cells. Collectively, it appears that glycoprotein expression by the embryo and the uterus is quite dynamic. This property is likely to have important consequences with regard to the cell-cell interactions that occur during implantation.

Introduction

The process by which mammalian embryos attach to and invade the uterine endometrium is both fascinating and complex.   From early conception until parturition, embryonal and maternal tissues must exist symbiotically without imposing detrimental effects on the other. It remains unclear why the immunologically-competent mother fails to reject the embryo in spite of histocompatibility differences. It also is unclear why the highly invasive trophoblast tissue of the embryo normally halts its progress within the endometrium although it clearly has the capacity to invade a wide range of tissues (16,32 and refs. cited within).   In this regard, the interesting feature of the uterus may not be that it supports embryo implantation, but that it has the unique ability to prevent and limit embryo invasion.

Whether or not the uterus will allow embryo attachment and invasion is determined by ovarian steroid hormone influences (50). Under the appropriate hormonal stimuli the uterus is transiently converted to a state receptive for embryo attachment. Following this receptive phase, the uterus returns to a non-receptive state until the steroid hormone levels decline and eventually reestablish themselves during the next ovarian cycle. This decline in steroid levels must occur before a receptive state can be reestablished. If embryo implantation occurs, the steroid hormone levels are maintained and the uterus remains non-receptive. The state of receptivity not only is characterized by marked differences in the ability of the uterus to support embryo attachment, but also in the ability of the uterus to regulate progression of various intraluminally-presented tumors (38-40,53,54). Consequently, the uterus appears to be an organ specially adapted to regulating the invasive potential of highly-invasive cell types in a hormone-dependent manner.

A sequence of events that occurs during the early phases of embryo implantation in rodents is described in Figure 1. Shortly after the embryo hatches from the zona pellucida it develops the ability to attach to various substrates. These substrates include various factors present in serum (57) as well as laminin (4,25,61), fibronectin (4,25,61), collagens (10,61), hyaluronic acid (11) and uterine epithelial cells (25,57). Histochemical studies have shown that the types of glycoconjugates expressed at the external surface of the blastocyst change as the embryo becomes attachment competent (23). Coordinated with the development of the embryo is the differentiation of the apical cell surface of the uterine epithelium. A number of histological studies have shown that glycoconjugate expression at this uterine cell surface also changes markedly as the uterus develops to a receptive state (1,2,23). Consequently, it has been suggested that cell surface glycoconjugates participate in or influence the interactions that occur between the blastocyst and the apical cell surface of the uterine epithelium (52).

As a consequence of embryo attachment as well as the hormonal status of the animal, the stromal tissue underlying the implantation site is triggered to differentiate in a process called the decidual cell response (28). The decidual tissue begins to express different cytoskeletal proteins as well as different extracellular matrix components (11,31,66,67). Many of these extracellular matrix components have been shown to support embryo outgrowth *in vitro* (4,10,11,25,61), a process believed to be analogous to embryo invasion *in vivo*. Finally, the embryo penetrates the deciduum and, curiously, then stops its invasion. Eventually, both trophoblastic and uterine cells will intermingle in hemochorial animals to form a placenta (8).

It is clear from the above description that one repetitive aspect of implantation-related processes is the alteration in expression of cell surface glycoconjugates. In this review, we will attempt to summarize our current knowledge of the factors influencing glycoprotein expression by peri-implantation stage embryos and uteri. Most of this discussion will focus upon information drawn from rodent model systems. This information will be put in the context of how such changes might impact upon the cell-cell interactions that occur during implantation.

Glycoprotein Expression by Peri-implantation Stage Embryos

A number of studies have described various aspects of glycoconjugate expression during the peri-implantation stage of embryo development. In addition to the histochemical studies referred to above, a number of biochemical studies have been performed. These studies have indicated changes in the patterns (44,49), and apparent biosynthetic rates (26,44,60) of glyco-proteins. Several studies have indicated that treatment of blastocysts with inhibitors of glycoprotein synthesis also inhibit embryo attachment and outgrowth formation (6,26,33,60). However, it is unclear whether these agents inhibit development by virtue of their effects on glycoprotein synthesis or by other, indirect effects. Elegant microanalytical techniques have shown that the activities of certain enzymes involved in glycoprotein assembly do not change markedly during the peri-implantation period (3). Consequently, it seems more likely that alterations in the expression of the corresponding classes of glycoproteins reflect changes in the expression of mRNA coding for glycoprotein core proteins.

Heparan sulfate proteoglycans (HSPGs) are a class of glycoproteins that have been shown to be expressed at the trophectodermal cell surface where they appear to participate in embryo attachment processes (25). As discussed above, the apparent rate of HSPG synthesis increases markedly during the peri-implantation stage. Moreover, inhibitors of HSPG synthesis inhibit embryo attachment to a variety of substrates, including uterine

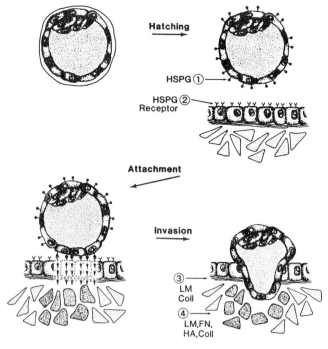

Figure 1. Model of mouse embryo implantation. Shortly after the embryo hatches from the zona pellucida it acquires the ability to attach to the uterine epithelial cell surface. One class of embryonic cell surface glycoproteins believed to be important in promoting attachment are the heparan sulfate proteoglycans (**HSPG**). HSPGs of the embryo cell surface are believed to interact with corresponding receptors on the apical cell surface of uterine epithelial cells. As a consequence of embryo attachment and the hormonal environment of the uterus signals are transduced from the embryo attachment site which initiate the decidual cell response in the underlying stroma. As the embryo invades the basal lamina and underlying stroma it encounters outgrowth-promoting glycoconjugates including laminin (**LM**), collagens (**COLL**), fibronectin (**FN**) and hyaluronic acid (**HA**). For details and references see text.

epithelial cells (26). It is not clear if HSPGs are necessary for embryo outgrowth formation since attachment is prerequisite for this process. Integrins and receptors recognizing RGD sequences in proteins are expressed by embryos and participate, at least, in outgrowth formation (5,10,25,61). Members of the integrin superfamily of cell adhesion proteins appear to interact with a number of the substrata that have been shown to support embryo attachment and outgrowth *in vitro*, e.g., fibronectin, laminin, and collagens. It is therefore possible that integrins mediate multiple aspects of embryo invasion *in utero*. More work must be done using probes specific to certain integrins to determine if members of this family of proteins are expressed differentially during development.

Expression of other cell adhesion-promoting glycoproteins has been studied in rodent blastocysts. For example, uvomorulin (E-cadherin) and cell CAM 105 begin to be expressed at the morula stage and continue to be expressed by peri-implantation stage blastocysts (62,65). However, by the peri-implantation stage these molecules are not present at the external surface of the trophectoderm and are therefore unavailable for initial embryo-uterine interactions. Certain collagens also are expressed by embryos at this stage and may be present on the external surface of the trophectoderm (36,56). In fact, it has been reported that embryo attachment proteins are particularly sensitive to collagenase digestion (55). Basement membrane components like laminin, entactin (nidogen) and HSPGs begin to be expressed during the 2-cell to morula stages of development (17,18). Furthermore, they continue to be expressed at the external surface of the trophectoderm at the peri-implantation stage (35,55,58). Electron microscopy of embryos at this stage fails to reveal any

109

evidence of an organized lamina at the external surface of the peri-implantation stage blastocyst (52,58). Nonetheless, the presence of multiple components of basal lamina indicate that this surface of the embryo has certain basement membrane-like characteristics at this stage.

Glycoprotein Expression by Uteri and Uterine Cell Types

Hormonal Factors. A variety of morphological studies have demonstrated that the expression of uterine glycoconjugates changes markedly during early pregnancy and in response to steroid hormones (1,2,23,52). In addition, biochemical studies indicate that the content of uterine glycoconjugates and relative metabolic rates of radioactive sugar incorporation into macromolecules changes under these conditions (21,22,35,41). In general, it appears that estrogens are potent stimulators of uterine glycoprotein synthesis. In contrast, progesterone alone does not appear to affect glycoprotein production; however, it strongly antagonizes estrogen action in this regard.

The activities of a number of enzymes involved in glycoprotein assembly and transfer have been examined. Some of these activities also appear to increase in response to estrogen treatment and are antagonized by progesterone (13,22,37,42,43). In other cases, the hormones have little effect on the activities of glycosyltransferases (13,22). Therefore, it appears that parts of the enzymatic machinery required for uterine glycoprotein assembly are expressed constitutively while other parts need to be amplified under conditions where glycoprotein production is enhanced.

A few studies have examined how the levels of substrates, e.g. sugar-nucleotides (21,22,24) and dolichol-linked saccharides (13), change in response to steroid hormones. In general, it appears that the hormones have little effect on the tissue concentrations of these compounds. These observations suggest that regulation of glycoprotein synthesis is not likely to be due to changes in substrate availability. It is possible that such substrates are compartmentalized within cells. Consequently, if steroid hormones influence this compartmentalization then redistribution of substrates could alter rates of glycoprotein synthesis.

The relative levels of mRNA coding for certain uterine glycoproteins increase greatly in response to estrogen (64). However, neither the relative mRNA levels nor the apparent rates of synthesis of the protein cores of other glycoproteins are stimulated by estrogen at the same time that sugar incorporation into these molecules is enhanced (27). Therefore, it seems that estrogen may not only promote uterine glycoprotein synthesis by inducing the expression of glycoprotein genes, but also by increasing the efficiency by which proteins are glycosylated. This differential glycosylation may affect the function or stability of these proteins (47).

As discussed above, the combined influences of estrogen and progesterone on uterine glycoprotein assembly are complex. While estrogen alone seems to be able to maximally promote many aspects of glycoprotein assembly, in many cases, progesterone alone has very little effect. Nonetheless, progesterone can dramatically attenuate the stimulatory effect of estrogen on glycoprotein assembly. In the case of N-linked glycoprotein assembly, this effect is not manifest at the level of the glycosylation apparatus nor at the level of the availability of substrates for glycosyltransferases (13,21,22). Thus, progesterone may modulate N-linked glycoprotein synthesis by regulating the expression of glycoprotein mRNA. In contrast, estrogen's primary influence on glycoprotein assembly may be at the level of the glycosylation apparatus.

Decidualization and Maturational Factors. Other factors influence uterine glycoprotein assembly as well. For instance, during the decidual response the stromal cells of the uterus begin expressing a battery of glycoconjugates at substantially higher levels (11,31,66,67). This response requires both an appropriate hormonal background (both progesterone and estrogen) as well as a stimulus. The stimulus is normally the embryo, but can be mimicked by the injection of oil or buffer into the uterine lumen (28).

Changes in glycoprotein expression do not occur for several days after administration of the decidual stimulus; however, increased synthesis of the non-protein-linked polysaccharide, hyaluronic acid, occurs almost immediately (11). Thus, some effects of the decidual response on glycoconjugate expression may be triggered by rapidly-acting processes occurring during this time, e.g. prostaglandin release (28,34). Other effects seem to develop comparatively slowly and may involve secondary responses to the decidual stimulus, e.g. increased transcription. With regard to the latter point, it appears that the increased expression of uterine extracellular matrix components that accompanies the decidual response is preceded by increased expression of the mRNA coding for these glycoproteins (19). The molecular signals responsible for increasing gene expression under these circumstances remain totally unknown.

It also has been reported that the immature uterus does not respond to estrogen in the same manner as the mature uterus (51). This point holds true for glycoprotein expression as well. N-Linked glycoprotein assembly is stimulated greatly by estrogen in both immature and mature mice (9,22). In mature mice, this effect is particularly evident in a subset of N-linked oligosaccharides, the lactosaminoglycans (LAGs; 21). LAGs not only are excellent indicators of estrogen action in uteri of mature mice, but also are major cell surface components of uterine epithelial cells and appear to participate in galactosyltransferase-dependent cell adhesion processes that occur among these cells (20). Although epithelial cells of immature mice synthesize LAGs, these oligosaccharides differ structurally in several respects, most notably by the fact that none are N-linked (9,20). In response to estrogen, immature epithelial cells display an enhanced ability to synthesize N-linked glycoproteins, but fail to synthesize N-linked LAGs. Consequently, additional maturational influences appear to be required to endow these cells with the ability to synthesize this interesting class of glycoproteins. Such influences may be derived from other hormones or stromal cells, but remain undefined at present.

Glycoprotein Expression by Uterine Epithelial Cells. Changes in the patterns of glycoprotein expression by uterine epithelial cells are of particular interest since it is the cell surface of these cells that mediates the initial phase of embryo-uterine attachment. Histochemical studies have shown that patterns of glycoconjugate expression at the luminal (apical) surfaces of these cells change during the conversion from a non-receptive to a receptive uterine state (1,2,52). One consistent observation is that the negative charge character of these surfaces decreases in the receptive state. Although relatively little molecular characterization of the cell surface of uterine epithelial cells has been described, one component of their apical cell surface appears to be HSPGs (45,46,63). In rats and mice, a transient rise in estrogen levels (nidatory estrogen) appears to be required to trigger production of a receptive uterine state (50). Morris and coworkers have suggested that estrogen stimulates a more rapid degradation of HSPGs (45,46). Consequently, it seems likely that one factor contributing to the decreased negative charge character of the apical surfaces of receptive cells is a decrease in the expression of HSPGs; however, this remains to be rigorously demonstrated.

Another consistent observation is that conversion to a receptive uterine state is accompanied by increased expression of N-acetylglucosaminyl and galactosyl residues (1,2,15). LAGs are a class of glycoproteins expressed at the cell surface of uterine epithelial cells that are polymers of alternating N-acetylglucosaminyl and galactosyl residues (29). As discussed above, LAGs have been shown to participate in cell adhesion processes that occur among uterine epithelial cells (20). Preliminary studies indicate that they also may be involved in aspects of embryo outgrowth formation *in vitro* (Jacobs and Carson, unpublished observations); however, attempts to detect LAGs at the lumenal surface of the uterus have not indicated that these glycoproteins are enriched at this area in receptive uteri (Dutt and Carson, unpublished studies). Nonetheless, LAGs can be found in the uterine lumen under various conditions (7). It is possible that subtle alterations in LAG structure influence the function of these oligosaccharides.

Some interesting points arise from the comparison of the metabolism of HSPGs and LAG-glycoproteins in uterine epithelial cells (14, 68). Both classes of glycoproteins require similar times (30 min) to move from the site of their core protein synthesis, the rough endoplasmic reticulum, to the site of complex oligosaccharide addition, the Golgi apparatus. At this point kinetic and metabolic differences arise. HSPGs move rapidly (6 ± 2 min) from the Golgi to the cell surface whereas LAG-glycoproteins require approximately 30 min to move between these compartments. It appears that both types of glycoproteins can be released from the cell surface by protease-mediated processes. However, while a large fraction the HSPGs are degraded by a chloroquine-sensitive pathway, presumably the lysosomes, LAG-glycoproteins appear to be nearly quantitatively secreted or released from the cell surface. HSPGs are relatively short-lived, exhibiting a metabolic half life of approximately 2 h. In contrast, LAG-glycoproteins are more stable, exhibiting a metabolic half life of approximately 6 h. For reference, the metabolic half life of bulk cell surface proteins is approximately 24 h (Carson, D.D., unpublished observations). Consequently, both types of glycoproteins "turn over" relatively rapidly by comparison to other proteins.

Collectively, these observations indicate that uterine epithelial cells are able to rapidly and differentially metabolize different cell surface components. Moreover, it appears that steroid hormones may influence these processes (21,45,46). These findings are consistent with the morphological studies demonstrating rapid changes in the composition of cell surface glycoconjugates that occur in response to steroid hormones and during the transition to a receptive uterine state (1,2,23,52).

An important aspect of epithelial cell structure is polarity (59). Epithelial cells, in general, organize their plasma membranes into distinct apical and basolateral domains. These domains have different compositions which reflect their different functions. A current problem of great interest in cell biology is how polarized cells target components to and regulate the distinct functions of their apical and basolateral plasma membrane domains. Uterine epithelial cells are no exception in this regard. It is clear that the apical and basal surfaces of uterine epithelial cells must support different processes. For example, the apical (lumenal) surface must support embryo attachment in a hormonally-regulated manner as well as mediate secretory activity into the uterine lumen. In contrast, the basal surface must maintain contact with the basal lamina and mediate interactions with stroma. The function of the apical surfaces of these cells has been approachable by monitoring lumenal secretions and luminally-disposed cell surface components; however, it has not been possible to study the corresponding aspects of the basolateral surfaces. The recent development of a culture system for polarized uterine epithelial cells is making it possible to study the separate functions of these plasma membrane domains *in vitro* (30). These studies have shown that these cells have distinctly different capacities for secreting proteins and glycoproteins from their apical versus basolateral surfaces (12,30). Recent studies also indicate that polarized cultures of uterine epithelial cells display estrogen responsiveness as well as secrete pro-staglandins with a marked basal preference (Jacobs, A., Julian, J., Decker, G.L., Carson, D.D. and Glasser, S.R., unpublished studies). Thus, it should be possible to use this system to determine if steroid hormones influence a variety of aspects of epithelial glycoprotein expression.

Glycoprotein Expression by Uterine Stromal Cells. In general, much less is known about regulation of glycoprotein expression by uterine stromal cells. Perhaps the most information in this regard has been derived from studies of the decidual response. A number of studies have shown that stromal cells begin to synthesize different glycoconjugates associated with cell adhesion processes as part of the decidual response. Notable examples include laminin (31,66,67), collagen type IV (66), a placental form of cadherin (48), as well as others (11). Some studies have indicated that the patterns of stromal proteoglycan expression are changed as part of the decidual response as well (66). A number of the glycoconjugates whose expression changes during the decidual response also have been shown to support embryo attachment and outgrowth *in vitro*. Examples of this include laminin (4,25,61), collagen type IV (10,61), hyaluronate (11) and fibronectin (4,25,61). Consequently, the changing pattern of stromal glycoprotein expression may have important influences on the ability of the embryo to invade the endometrium.

A number of factors including steroid hormones and prostaglandins have been implicated as important mediators of the decidual response (28). Nonetheless, very little is known about the factors controlling this differentiative response of the uterus with regard to the changing pattern of glycoprotein expression. Appropriate molecular probes are available to study glycoprotein expression in this system; however, the decidual response seems to occur spontaneously in stromal cells cultured *in vitro* (31,66). Consequently, it has been difficult to study the factors controlling this process. Clearly, it is possible to control the decidual response in utero (28). Thus, it may be feasible to determine which factors are responsible for activating expression of certain stromal glycoproteins. Nonetheless, this approach seems unworkable when it comes to studying the role that genetic factors, e.g. steroid response elements, associated with glycoprotein expression play in this process. For such studies, it would be desirable to work with isolated stromal cell cultures. With this approach, stromal cells could be transfected with reporter genes coupled to potential regulatory sequences of the glycoprotein gene of interest. Transfected cells would then be treated with agents known to trigger the decidual response and the effects on reporter gene expression examined. In this way, one could determine if "decidual response elements" occurred in glycoprotein genes. It first may be necessary to develop a reproducible, controllable model of the decidual response *in vitro* before detailed molecular studies of this aspect of stromal cell differentiation can be performed.

Conclusion

The patterns of expression of cell surface and extracellular matrix glycoproteins change markedly in both embryos and uterine cells during the peri-implantation stage of development. A number of the molecules involved in these changes have been shown to have the capacity to function in cell adhesion processes that occur among embryos and various uterine cell types. Regulation of the expression of glycoproteins by embryos appears to be under developmental control. In the uterus glycoprotein expression changes in response to a number of factors. Changes in the pattern of glycoprotein expression include effects on the glycosylation apparatus as well as transcriptional effects on glycoprotein mRNA expression. These uterine processes are influenced strongly by the hormonal milieu, the sexual maturity of the animal, the state of cell polarity in the case of epithelial cells as well as by uterine cell-cell interactions that are, as yet, poorly understood.

Acknowledgments

We are grateful to M. Farach-Carson, M. Valdizan, J. D. Farrar, and L. Rohde for their many helpful discussions and their critical readings of this manuscript. We acknowledge the support of NIH grant HD 25235 and American Cancer Society Grant BC-503 in these studies. We thank Ms. Ellen Madson and Mrs. Harriette Young for their excellent typing. N.R. was supported by NIH grant HD 25235 and A.L.J. was supported by American Cancer Society grant BC-503.

References

1. Anderson, T. L., Hoffman L. H., Alterations in epithelial glycocalyx of rabbit uteri during early pseudopregnancy and pregnancy, and following ovariectomy, Amer. J. Anat. 171:321 (1984).
2. Anderson, T. L., Olson, G. E., Hoffman, L., Stage-specific alterations in the apical membrane glycoproteins of endometrial epithelial cells related to implantation in rabbits, Biol. Reprod., 34:701 (1986).
3. Armant, D. R., Kaplan, H. A., and Lennarz, W. J., N-Linked glycoprotein biosynthesis in the developing mouse embryo, Dev. Biol., 113:228 (1986).

4. Armant, D. R., Kaplan, H. A., and Lennarz, W. J., Fibronectin and laminin promote *in vitro* attachment and outgrowth of mouse blastocysts, Dev. Biol., 116:519 (1986).

5. Armant, D. R., Kaplan, H. A., Mover, H., and Lennarz, W. J., The effect of hexapeptides on attachment and outgrowth of mouse embryo *in vitro*: Evidence for the involvement of the cell recognition tripeptide Arg-Gly-Asp, Proc. Natl. Acad. Sci. USA, 83:6751 (1986).

6. Atienza-Samols, S. B., Pine, S. R., and Sherman, M. I., Effects of tunicamycin upon glycoprotein synthesis and development of early mouse embryos, Dev. Biol., 79:19 (1980).

7. Babiarz, B. and Hathaway, H. J., Hormonal control of the expression of antibody-defined lactosaminoglycans in the mouse uterus, Biol. Reprod., 39:699 (1988).

8. Benirschke, K., Placentation, J. Exp. Zool., 228:385 (1983).

9. Carson, D. D. and Tang, J. P., Estrogen induces N-linked glycoprotein expression by immature mouse uterine epithelial cells, Biochem., 28:8116 (1990).

10. Carson, D. D., Tang, J. P., and Gay, S., Collagens support embryo attachment and outgrowth *in vitro*: Effects of the Arg-Gly-Asp sequence, Dev. Biol., 127:368 (1988).

11. Carson, D. D., Dutt, A., and Tang, J. P., Glycoconjugate synthesis during early pregnancy: hyaluronate synthesis and function, Dev. Biol., 120:228 (1987).

12. Carson, D. D., Tang, J. P., Julian, J., and Glasser, S. R., Vectorial secretion of proteoglycans by polarized rat uterine epithelial cells, J. Cell Biol., 107:2425 (1988).

13. Carson, D. D., Tang, J. P., and Hu, G., Estrogen influences dolichylphosphate distribution among glycolipid pools in mouse uteri, Biochemistry, 26:1598 (1987).

14. Carson, D. D., Wilson, O. F., and Dutt, A., Glycoconjugate expression and interactions at the cell surface of mouse uterine epithelial cells and peri-implantation-stage embryos, Troph. Res. 4:211 (1990).

15. Chavez, D. J. and Anderson, T. L., The glycocalyx of the mouse uterine epithelium during estrus, early pregnancy, the peri-implantation period and delayed implantation. I. The acquisition of Ricinus communis I binding sites during pregnancy, Biol. Reprod., 32:1135 (1985).

16. Cowell, T. P., Implantation and development of mouse eggs transferred to the uteri of non-progestational mice, J. Reprod. Fertil., 19:239 (1969).

17. Dziadek, M., Fujiwara, S., Paulsson, M., and Timpl, R., Immunological characterization of basement membrane types of heparan sulfate proteoglycan, EMBO J., 4:905 (1985).

18. Dziadek, M. and Timpl, R., Expression of nidogen and laminin in basement membranes during mouse embryogenesis and in teratocarcinoma cells, Dev. Biol., 111:372 (1985).

19. Dutt, A., Cooper, J., Stewart, S. L., Farrar, J. D., and Carson, D. D., Regulation of extracellular matrix expression during uterine decidualization [abstract] J. Cell Biol., 107:4538 (1988).

20. Dutt, A., Tang, J. P., and Carson, D. D., Lactosaminoglycans are involved in uterine epithelial cell adhesion *in vitro*, Dev. Biol., 119:27 (1987).

21. Dutt, A., Tang, J. P., and Carson, D. D., Estrogen preferentially stimulates lactosaminoglycan-containing oligosaccharide synthesis in mouse uteri, J. Biol. Chem., 263:2270 (1988).

22. Dutt, A., Tang, J. P., Welply, J. K., and Carson, D. D., Regulation of N-linked glycoprotein assembly in uteri by steroid hormones, Endocrinology, 118:661 (1986).

23. Enders, A. C. and Schlafke, S., Surface coats of the mouse blastocyst and uterus during the preimplantation period, Anat. Rec., 180:31 (1974).

24. Endo, M. and Yosizawa, Z., Hormonal effects on sugar-nucleotides in rabbit uteri, Arch. Biochem. Biophys., 127:585 (1968).

25. Farach, M. C., Tang, J. P., Decker, G. L., and Carson, D. D., Heparan/heparan sulfate is involved in attachment and spreading of mouse embryos *in vitro*, Dev. Biol., 123:401 (1987).

26. Farach, M. C., Tang, J. P., Decker, G. L., and Carson, D. D., Differential effects of p-nitrophenyl-D-xylosides on mouse blastocysts and uterine epithelial cells, Biol. Reprod., 39:443 (1988).

27. Carson, D.D., Farrar, J. D., Laidlaw and Wright, D.A., Selective activation of 5the N-glycosylation apparatus in uteri by estrogen, J. Biol. Chem., 265:2947 (1990).

28. Finn, C. A., Implantation, menstruation and inflammation, Biol. Rev., 61:313 (1986).

29. Fukuda, M., Cell surface glycoconjugates as onco-differentiation markers in hematopoietic cells, Biochim. Biophys. Acta, 780:119 (1985).

30. Glasser, S. R., Julian, J., Decker, G. L., Tang, J. P., and Carson, D. D., Development of morphological and functional polarity in primary cultures of immature rat uterine epithelial cells, J. Cell Biol., 107:2409 (1988).

31. Glasser, S. R., Lampelo, S., Munir, M. I., and Julian, J., Expression of desmin, laminin and fibronectin during *in situ* differentiation (decidualization) of rat uterine stromal cells. Differentiation, 35:132 (1987).

32. Gurchot, C., The trophoblast theory of cancer (John Beard, 1857-1924) revisited, Oncology, 31:310 (1969).

33. Iwakura, Y. and Nozaki, M., Effect of tunicamycin on preimplantaton mouse embryos: prevention of molecular differentiation during blastocyst formation, Dev. Biol., 112:124 (1985).

34. Kennedy, T., The role of prostaglandins in endometrial vascular changes at implantation, In: *Cellular and Molecular Aspects of Implantation*, S. R. Glasser and R. W. Bullock, (eds.), New York, Plenum Press (1981), pp. 349.

35. Lambadarios, C., Hastings, C., Abo-Darub, J., and Cooke, I. D., Steroid effects on human endometrial glycoprotein synthesis, J. Reprod. Fertil., 46:383 (1976).

36. Leivo, I., Vaheri, A., Timpl, R., and Wartiovaara, J., Appearance and distribution of collagens and laminins in the early mouse embryo, Dev. Biol., 76:100 (1980).

37. Nelson, J. D., Jato-Rodriguez, J. J., and Mookerjea, S., Effect of ovarian hormones on glycosyltransferase activities in the endometrium of ovariectomized rats, Arch. Biochem. Biophys., 169:181 (1975).

38. Maharajan, P. and Maharajan, V., Behavioral pattern of tumour cells in mouse uterus, Gynecol. Obstet. Inves., 21:32 (1986).

39. Maharajan, P., Rosato, F., and Maharajan, V., Response of mouse embryos to tumour extract treatment, Gynecol. Obstet. Invest., 23:208 (1987).

40. Maharajan, P., Rosato, F., Mirabella, N., Pelayalli, G., and Maharajan, V., Influence of mouse uterus on the metastatic patterns of tumour cells, Canc. Lett., 43:33 (1988).

41. Munakata, H., Isemura, M., Aikawa, J., Kodama, C., and Yosizawa, Z., Changes of glycosaminoglycan composition of uterine myometrium of rabbit induced by female sex steroids, Tohoku. J. Exp. Med., 147:77 (1985).

42. Munakata, H., Isemura, M., and Yosizawa, Z., Effects of female hormones on the activity of 3'-phosphoadenylylsulphate: desulphated heparan sulfate sulphotransferase in the endometrium of rabbit uterus, Int. J. Biochem., 17:1077 (1985).

43. Munakata, H., Isemura, M., and Yosizawa, Z., Enzymatic sulfation of exogenous high molecular weight glycopeptides by microsomal fraction of the rabbit uterine endometrium, J. Biol. Chem., 260: 6851 (1985).

44. Muramatsu, T., Developmentally regulated expression of cell surface carbohydrates during mouse embryogenesis, J. Cell. Biochem., 36:1 (1988).

45. Morris, J. E., Potter, S. W., and Gaza-Bulesco, G., Estradiol induces an accumulation of free heparan sulfate glycosaminoglycan chains in uterine epithelium, Endocrinology, 122:242 (1988).

46. Morris, J. E., Potter, S. W., and Gaza-Bulesco, G., Estradiol-stimulated turnover of heparan sulfate proteoglycan in mouse uterine epithelium, J. Biol. Chem., 263:4712 (1988).

47. Olden, K., Parent, J. B., and White, S. L., Carbohydrate moieties of glycoproteins, a reevaluation of their function, Biochim. Biophys. Acta, 650:209 (1982).

48. Nose, A. and Takeichi, M., A novel cadherin adhesion molecule: Its expression patterns associated with implantation and organogenesis of mouse embryos, J. Cell Biol., 103:2649 (1986).

49. Pinsker, M. C. and Mintz, B., Change in cell-surface glycoproteins of mouse embryos before implantation, Proc. Natl. Acad. Sci. USA, 70:1645 (1973).
50. Psychoyos, A., Hormonal control of ovum implantation, Vit. Horm., 31:201 (1973).
51. Quarmby V.E. and Korach K.S., The influence of 17-β-estradiol on patterns of cell division in the uterus, Endocrinology, 114:694 (1984).
52. Schlafke, S. and Enders, A. C., Cellular basis of interaction between trophoblast and uterus at implantation, Biol. Reprod., 12:41 (1975).
53. Schleich, A. B., Frick, M., and Mayer, A., Patterns of invasive growth *in vitro*. Human decidua graviditatis confronted with established human cell lines and primary human explants, J. Natl. Canc. Inst., 56:221 (1976).
54. Schlesinger, M., Uterus of rodents as site for manifestation of transplantation immunity against transplantable tumors, J. Natl. Canc. Inst., 28:927 (1962).
55. Sherman, M. I. and Atienza-Samols, S. B., *In vitro* studies on the adhesiveness of mouse blastocysts, In: *Human Fertilization*, H. Ludwig and P. Taiber, (eds.), PGS, Boston (1978), pp. 179.
56. Sherman, M. I., Gay, R., Gay, S., and Miller, E. J., Association of collagen with preimplantation mouse embryos, Dev. Biol., 74:270 (1980).
57. Sherman, M. I. and Salomon, D. S., The relationship between the early mouse embryo and its environment, In: *Developmental Biology of Reproduction*, C. L. Markert and J. Papaconstantinou, (eds.), New York, Academic Press (1975) pp. 277.
58. Sherman, M. I. and Wudl, L. R., The implanting mouse blastocyst, In: *The Cell Surface of Animal Development*, G. Poste and F. R. Nicolson, (eds.), North Holland Publ., Amsterdam (1976), p. 81.
59. Simons, K. and Fuller, S. D., Cell surface polarity in epithelia, Ann. Rev. Cell Biol., 1:243 (1985).
60. Surani, M. A. H., Glycoprotein synthesis and inhibition of protein glycosylation by tunicamycin in preimplantation embryos: influence on compaction and trophoblast adhesion, Cell, 18:217 (1979).
61. Sutherland, A. E., Calarco, P. G., and Damsky, C. H., Expression and function of cell surface extracellular matrix receptors in mouse blastocyst attachment and outgrowth, J. Cell Biol., 106:1331 (1988).
62. Svalander, P. C., Odin, P., Nilsson, B. O., and Obrink, B., Trophectoderm surface expression of the cell adhesion molecule cell-CAM 105 on rat blastocysts, Develop., 100:653 (1987).
63. Tang, J. P., Julian, J., Glasser, S. R., and Carson, D. D., Heparan sulfate proteoglycan synthesis and metabolism by mouse uterine epithelial cells cultured *in vitro*, J. Biol. Chem., 262:12832 (1987).
64. Teng, C. T., Pentecost, B. T., Chen, Y. H., Newbold, R. R., Eddy, E. M., and McLachlan, J. A., Lactotransferrin gene expression in the mouse uterus and mammary gland, Endocrinology, 124:992 (1989).
65. Vestweber, D., Gossler, A., Boller, K., and Kemler, R., Expression and distribution of cell adhesion molecule uvomorulin in preimplantation embryos, Dev. Biol., 124:451 (1987).
66. Wewer, V. M., Damjanov, A., Weiss, J., Liotta, L. A., and Damjanov, I., Mouse endometrial stromal cells produce basement membrane components, Differentiation, 32:49 (1986).
67. Wu, T. C., Wan, Y. J., Chung, A. E., and Damjanov, I., Immunohistochemical localization of entactin and laminin in mouse embryos and fetuses, Dev. Biol., 100:496 (1983).
68. Duff, A. and Carson, D.D., Lactosaminoglycan assembly, cell surface expression, and release by mouse uterine epithelial cells, J. Biol. Chem., 265:430 (1990).

Questions

Dr. Bigsby: Dan, if I can remember my reproductive biology correctly, there is a difference between attachment and implantation, obviously. But also, within the uterus there is a difference in location, that is, mesometrial versus antimesometrial. Have you addressed that?

Dr. Carson: We have not addressed that and that is a very important point. There a variety of other criteria used to decide if a molecule is involved in embryo attachment. One that I discussed was regulation by steroid hormones. Another issue that you bring up is that it would have to be expressed or at least available on the antimesometrial side. Another criteria is that embryos only attach at their mural trophectoderm, they don't attach at their polar trophectoderm, so there should be a sidedness in the embryo as well with regard to the molecules involved in the attachment process. We haven't addressed that yet because we don't have the tools to address that with, but we need to address it if any of this is to mean anything in terms of implantation. That's a good question.

10

Uterine-conceptus Interactions During the Peri-implantation Period

F.W. Bazer
Departments of Animal Science and Pediatrics
University of Florida
Gainesville,   Florida 32611

Summary

Interactions between the conceptus and endometrium of sheep and pigs are essential for establishment and maintenance of pregnancy. In pigs, estrogen-induced redirection of secretion of prostaglandin $F_{2\alpha}$ (PGF) into the uterine lumen (exocrine secretion) is antiluteolytic, while sheep conceptuses secrete ovine trophoblast protein-1 which inhibits episodic secretion of PGF from the endometrium which is required for luteolysis. These antiluteolytic mechanisms insure maintenance of functional corpora lutea and secretion of progesterone which stimulates endometrial secretion of factors required to support the developing embryo/conceptus. These secretions include nutrients, as well as proteins that serve as enzymes, transport proteins, and regulatory proteins essential for establishment and maintenance of a successful pregnancy.

Introduction

Pregnancy is established and maintained in response to interactions between the conceptus (embryo/fetus and its associated membranes and fluids) and the endometrium. This chapter includes information describing early development of the sheep and pig conceptuses, events associated with establishment of intimate contact between the conceptus and uterine endometrium and conceptus signals affecting the maternal system which allow maintenance of an intrauterine environment supportive of pregnancy.

Discussion

Conceptus Development

Information presented in this section has been reviewed extensively (13). Pig and sheep embryos fail to develop beyond the early blastocyst stage if confined to the oviduct. The absence of factors essential for further embryonic development or the presence of embryotoxic factors may be responsible for this phenomenon. Pig embryos begin intrauterine migration as early as Day 9 and migration and spacing is terminated by Days 11 to 12 when the blastocysts elongate. Intrauterine migration and spacing of blastocysts appears to be modulated by peristaltic contractions of the myometrium stimulated by products secreted by developing blastocysts, e.g., estrogens, histamines and prostaglandins. Transuterine migration of blastocysts is rare in monovulatory ewes, but common following multiple ovulations from the same ovary. Intrauterine migration and spacing of sheep blastocysts also ends on Days 12 to 13 when they undergo elongation and initiate placentation.

Pig embryos hatch from the zona pellucida between Days 6 and 7, have a diameter of 2 to 6 mm by Day 10 and undergo morphological transition from large spheres (10 to 15 mm diameter) to tubular (1 to 2 mm x 15 to 50 mm) and filamentous forms (1 mm x 100 to 200 mm) between Days 10 and 12. Between Days 10 and 12, conceptuses elongate at a rate of 30 to 45 mm/h; primarily by cellular remodeling and not cellular hyperplasia (50). However, continued growth and elongation of the conceptuses to 800 to 1000 mm length by Day 15 does involve cellular hyperplasia. Associated with morphological elongation of conceptuses is initiation of estrogen secretion, a marked increase in free calcium in the uterine lumen and significant increases in intraluminal prostaglandins (PG) $F_{2\alpha}$ (PGF) and PGE_2 (PGE), as well as plasminogen activator, hyaluronic acid and hyaluronidase which are associated with tissue remodelling. The mechanism(s) responsible for elongation of pig conceptuses is unknown; however, alterations in the actin cytoskeleton and possibly other cytoskeletal components are involved (4).

Sheep blastocysts are spherical on Day 10 (0.4 mm) and elongate to filamentous conceptuses by Days 12 (1.0 x 33 mm), 14 (1 x 68 mm) and 15 (1 x 150 to 190 mm). Elongation continues until the trophoblast extends through the uterine body and into the contralateral uterine horn by Days 16 to 17 of pregnancy. Elongation of pig and sheep conceptuses involves the trophoblast and does not require the embryonic disc in sheep (43).

During expansion and elongation of pig and sheep conceptuses, mesoderm from the embryonic disc migrates between the trophectoderm and endoderm. Associated with outgrowth of the embryonic mesoderm is the initiation of secretion of proteins, prostaglandins and steroids by the conceptus. This will be discussed in more detail later in this chapter. This mesodermal layer divides and combines with trophectoderm to form the chorion and with endoderm to form the yolk sac. The mesoderm also contributes to formation of the amnion and allantois which are essential for histotrophic and hematotrophic nutrition of the embryo/fetus.

Pregnancy Factors

An "early pregnancy factor" (EPF), presumably a protein, is released from the pregnant uterus during the preimplantation period and affects maternal lymphocytes (see 89). EPF in serum is believed to be from maternal tissue and to represent two components, EPF-A and EPF-B. EPF-A is produced by the oviduct during estrus, activated by EPF-B and binds to lymphocytes. EPF-B or "ovum factor" is released from the ovary, presumably in response to a "signal" from the fertilized ovum. Results of studies of EPF with rodents and humans are controversial, while the presence of EPF in sheep and pigs has not been established.

Another preimplantation response, which may be related to EPF (63), is an increase in platelet activating factor (a family of acetylated glycerophospholipids known to release histamine from platelets, PAF) on Day 2 of pregnancy in mice (96). Reduced platelet numbers, thrombocytopenia, occurs within 3h after transfer of fertilized ova to pseudopregnant recipients and is correlated (r = + 0.86) with the number of embryos transferred. O'Neill (96) reported that PAF is responsible for thrombocytopenia, that 16-cell mouse embryos release PAF into culture medium and that parallel effects are induced with 1-O-alkyl-2-acetyl-sn-glycero (3) phosphocholine (PAF-acether), a potent PAF analog. Data are not available to indicate the presence or absence of PAF in conceptuses of large domestic animals.

PAF may not be essential for survival of preimplantation embryos in mice, but it increases their metabolic activity, e.g., increases incorporation of leucine and utilization of glucose and lactate (97). PAF also increases capillary permeability and dilation of the vascular bed to increase substrate delivery to implantation sites (63). Treatment of mice with PAF antagonists either reduces (115,116) or has no effect (80) on implantation rate, while in rats PAF antagonists almost completely inhibit implantation (1,2). In addition, administration of PAF to intact estrous mice results in appearance of EPF in serum (63). Differential transport of fertilized embryos of horses, bats and rats from the oviduct to uterus may be due to the release of PAF from fertilized, but not nonfertilized ova (63). If true, this would represent the first critical interaction between the zygote and endometrium affecting embryonic survival; subprimate embryos confined to the oviductal environment do not develop beyond the blastocyst stage (see 13).

Antiluteolytic Factors From Conceptuses of Pigs and Sheep

Conceptuses of domestic animals produce proteins, steroids and prostaglandins which serve as regulatory molecules affecting establishment and maintenance of pregnancy. An essential "signal" must be produced at a precise time and in adequate amounts to allow maintenance of corpus luteum (CL) function and continued production of progesterone, i.e., maternal recognition of pregnancy (107). Maintenance of progesterone production by CL is essential for maintenance of an intrauterine environment that will support conceptus development.

The endometrium secretes prostaglandin-F (PGF),the uterine luteolytic factor, responsible for regression of CL in sheep and pigs. Conceptuses of sheep and pigs produce proteins, steroids and prostaglandins during early pregnancy which may protect CL from luteolytic effects of PGF. Conceptus secretory products of pigs and sheep do not inhibit uterine production of PGF, but alter the pattern of secretion of PGF to one which is not luteolytic.

Homogenates of sheep conceptuses would, when infused into the uterine lumen, but not the utero-ovarian venous drainage, lead to longer interestrous intervals in ewes (86,87). Homogenates of sheep conceptuses do not contain either chorionic gonadotrophin-like or prolactin-like proteins (35). Therefore, the question of whether sheep conceptuses secrete a protein(s) that might function as an antiluteolytic agent was addressed by culturing Day 16 sheep conceptuses in the presence of radiolabelled amino acids and analyzing proteins released into the culture medium by two dimensional gel electrophoresis (2D-PAGE) and fluorography. The major protein detected by 2D-PAGE and Sephadex G 200 gel filtration had estimated Mr of 20,000 to 25,000 and pI values between 5.0 and 5.5 (128). This protein was initially referred to as protein X (53) and later as ovine trophoblast protein-1 (oTP-1)(55), because it is the first major protein secreted by mononuclear cells of ovine trophectoderm.

Sheep conceptuses secrete oTP-1 between Days 10 and 21 of pregnancy. The following are characteristics of oTP-1 (see 16,19): (1) molecular weight of about 19,000 and pI values of 5.3 to 5.7; (2) no carbohydrate moiety; (3) secreted by trophectoderm and taken up by endometrial surface epithelium and superficial glandular epithelium; (4) does not stimulate progesterone secretion by luteal tissue; (5) inhibits cAMP, but has no direct effect on cGMP and inositol phospholipid turnover in endometrial tissue; (6) strongly amplifies endometrial secretion of at least five proteins for which functions have not been determined; (7) high amino acid sequence homology with interferons of the alpha-II ($IFN\alpha_{II}$) class (26,66,117); (8) antiviral activity equivalent to that of recombinant human and bovine $IFN\alpha_I$ (100) and (9) immunosuppressive activity (94). oTP-1 is the only antiluteolytic paracrine hormone secreted by the sheep conceptus which inhibits pulsatile secretion of PGF by the endometrium to allow maternal recognition of pregnancy (123).

Endometrium of cyclic ewes releases PGF in a pulsatile manner between Days 14 and 17 of the cycle and about 5 episodes of PGF in 24 h are required for luteolysis (132,133). It has been proposed that estradiol from ovarian follicles induces endometrial oxytocin receptors and that oxytocin stimulates uterine secretion of luteolytic pulses of PGF (79). Oxytocin from the posterior pituitary and CL is released coincidentally to control pulsatile secretion of PGF by uterine endometrium (41,65). The pattern of release of oxytocin is not different between cyclic and pregnant ewes (65); however, oxytocin receptor numbers are significantly reduced or absent in pregnant compared to cyclic ewes (41,79,105).

Fincher *et al.* (38) infused total sheep conceptus secretory proteins (oCSP) or serum proteins into each uterine horn of cyclic ewes between Days 12 and 14 and injected 0.5 mg estradiol i.v. on Day 14 followed by 10 I.U. oxytocin on Day 15 to determine effects of oCSP on uterine production of PGF after the uterus had been stimulated by the hormones essential for luteolysis, i.e., estradiol and oxytocin. oCSP inhibited uterine production of PGF in response to both oestradiol and oxytocin. Pregnant ewes also fail to respond to the luteolytic effects associated with estradiol (38,73) and oxytocin (36). Comparison of antiluteolytic effects of intrauterine infusions of highly purified oTP-1, oCSP, oCSP minus oTP-1 and serum proteins indicated that oTP-1 alone had an antiluteolytic effect equivalent to that of oCSP (123). Infusion of oCSP minus oTP-1 or serum proteins did not inhibit uterine production of PGF in response to estradiol and oxytocin and did not extend the interestrous interval. Therefore, oTP-1 appears to be the only antiluteolytic protein secreted by sheep conceptuses.

How does oTP-1 inhibit oxytocin-induced episodic release of PGF from the endometrium of pregnant ewes? oTP-1 does not bind to the oxytocin receptor (see 19) or inhibit oxytocin-induced turnover of phosphatidylinositol (PI) in endometrium if oxytocin receptors are present on endometrial membranes (124, 125). In fact, PI turnover (125) and secretion of PGF (124) increased when endometrium was exposed to oTP-1 and then oxytocin. Induction of the antiviral state by IFNα in some cells requires stimulation of the cyclooxygenase system (101); an effect which could explain increased PI turnover and PGF production in endometrium exposed to oTP-1 and then oxytocin.

The temporal sequence of events associated with estradiol-induced luteolysis in ewes has been described (64). Administration of estradiol to ewes on Days 9 and 10 of the estrous cycle resulted in: (1) increased numbers of endometrial receptors for oxytocin within 12 h; (2) increased oxytocin-induced PI turnover at 24 h; (3) episodic secretion of PGF at 35 ± 3 h; (4) declining concentrations of progesterone in plasma at 42 ± 3 h and (5) estrous behavior at 69 ± 7 h. Secretion of oxytocin by the CL was first detected at 26 ± 3 h or about 9 h prior to detection of luteolytic pulses of PGF. Our hypothesis is that oTP-1 acts on the uterine endometrium to prevent synthesis of oxytocin receptors and thus rendering the endometrium incapable of releasing PGF in a pulsatile manner. Results of recent experiments support that hypothesis. First, PI turnover (83) and PGF secretion (124) in response to oxytocin are inhibited when endometrium of cyclic ewes is exposed to oTP-1 on Days 12 through 14. oTP-1 may inhibit synthesis and/or recycling of endometrial receptors for oxytocin, e.g., INFα can inhibit synthesis, turnover and movement of receptors within membranes (37,120). Endometrial receptors for oxytocin are present in increasing concentrations between Days 14 and 16 of the estrous cycle, but remain low or undetectable in pregnant ewes during this period (41,79). Temporal changes in endometrial receptors for progesterone during the estrous cycle and early pregnancy have not been described. However, estrogen receptor concentrations in endometrium are significantly lower in pregnant ewes on Days 9, 13 and 15, but not Day 11 (39). Since estradiol is responsible for induction of endometrial receptors for oxytocin (64,79), lower concentrations of estrogen receptors in early pregnancy may be part of the conceptus-mediated antiluteolytic mechanism. Reports of effects of IFNα on steroid receptors in endometrium indicate either no effect (68) or a stimulatory effect (34). Further research is required to determine the mechanism whereby oTP-1 exerts its antiluteolytic effect(s) on sheep endometrium.

Concentrations of PGE in utero-ovarian vein plasma of pregnant ewes increases markedly on Days 13 and 14 and PGE may play a luteal protective role (108). There is a high PGE:PGF ratio in the uterine lumen of pregnant ewes which may reflect the fact that conceptuses produce primarily PGE and alter uterine production of prostaglandins.

The theory of maternal recognition of pregnancy in pigs has been reviewed extensively (see 15,16,19). The assumptions are that PGF is the uterine luteolysin and that estrogens secreted by the conceptuses are antiluteolytic. The theory is that PGF is secreted in an endocrine direction (toward the uterine vasculature) in cyclic gilts and transported to the CL to exert its luteolytic effect. However, in pregnant pigs, the direction of secretion of PGF is exocrine (into the uterine lumen) where it is sequestered to exert its biological effects in utero and/or be metabolized to prevent luteolysis. Secretion of other components of histotroph, e.g., uteroferrin is also maintained in an exocrine direction in pregnant pigs (28).

Using an endometrial perifusion system (74), it was confirmed that endometrium from cyclic pigs secretes PGF primarily from the myometrial side (endocrine) and that endometrium from pregnant gilts secrete PGF primarily from the luminal side (exocrine)(57). The transition from endocrine to exocrine secretion occurs between Days 10 and 12 of pregnancy which is temporally associated with initiation of estrogen secretion by elongating pig conceptuses. Estrogens, secreted by the conceptus or injected, induce a transient release of calcium into the uterine lumen within 12 h. When endometrium from Day 14 cyclic gilts is treated in the perifusion device with the calcium ionophore A23187 (an inducer of calcium cycling by epithelium) secretion of PGF in the exocrine mode increased. These results suggest that induction of calcium cycling across endometrial epithelium is associated with redirection of secretion of PGF toward the uterine lumen (81).

Interactions between estrogen and prolactin enhance uterine secretory activity previously associated with estrogen-induced calcium cycling (131). Endometrium from Day 11 cyclic gilts treated with estradiol responded to prolactin by switching secretion of PGF from an endocrine to an exocrine direction; however, this effect of prolactin was not detected if gilts were not treated with estradiol (81). Estradiol induces endometrial receptors for prolactin in pigs (130) which may allow prolactin to induce calcium cycling across the epithelium and redirect secretion of PGF into the uterine lumen.

Estradiol must be administered to gilts on Day 11 and Days 14-16 to obtain interestous intervals of greater than 60 days, whereas a single injection of estradiol on either Day 9.5, 11, 12.5, 14, 15.5 or 14-16 resulted in interestrous intervals of about 30 days (51). This suggests that two phases of estradiol, similar to that produced by conceptuses on Days 11-13 and Days 15 to 30, are necessary for prolonged secretion of PGF in an exocrine direction. Estradiol may induce receptors for maternal hormones, e.g., prolactin, or conceptus secretory proteins, which influence exocrine secretion of PGF. The first estrogen signal may induce those receptors and the second estrogen signal may be for replenishment of those receptors. Administration of estradiol on Day 9 advances the uterine secretory response in pregnant gilts which leads to conceptus death by Day 16 (88). An explanation for this "induced" conceptus death is not available, but it may result from ansynchrony between the conceptus and uterine environment (88).

Pig conceptuses secrete two major classes of proteins with Mr of 20,000 to 25,000 (pI values of 5.6 to 6.2) and 35,000 to 50,000 (pI values of 8.2 to 9.0) between Days 10.5 and 18 of gestation (54). Pig conceptus secretory proteins (pCSP) recovered from culture medium of Day 15 conceptuses include a protein(s) with antiviral activity (20,30,62,82). Intrauterine infusion of 4 mg pCSP plus 4 mg serum proteins (SP) or 8 mg SP twice daily between Days 12 and 15 after i.m. administration of 1 mg estradiol on Day 11 of the estrous cycle had no effect on interestrous interval or temporal changes in concentrations of progesterone in plasma (60). Rather, pCSP-treatment stimulated uterine production of PGF (measured as PGFM) and PGE. These results indicate that pCSP are not antiluteolytic, but play other roles in early pregnancy.

Estradiol may affect maintenance of CL by acting directly on luteal cells to increase receptors for luteinizing hormone (LH, 48) and/or prolactin (23); however, this has not been clearly established. Maintenance of CL occurs in hysterectomized pigs because the source of PGF is removed and basal LH support is available. A luteotrophic hormone, produced by the conceptus, should have a systemic effect; however, the pig requires the presence of at least two conceptuses in each uterine horn to establish pregnancy. Maternal recognition of pregnancy in pigs probably results from local antiluteolytic effects of estradiol of conceptus origin on the endometrium to allow PGF to be sequestered in the uterine lumen.

Retinol binding protein is a major component of pCSP secreted between Days 10 and 16 of pregnancy (61) and it is also secreted by endometrial epithelium in response to progesterone (3). Retinoids affect gene transcription (29), cellular differentiation and proliferation (104), epithelial cell integrity and function and steroidogenesis (see 9), hematopoiesis and immune cell function (5) and interferon production (21,22). Each of these functions can be related to important events in pregnancy.

Endometrial Secretions in Pigs and Sheep

Species having conceptuses with noninvasive implantation depend upon secretions of endometrial epithelium for most, if not all of pregnancy (see 14,102). Peptides and proteins which serve as nutrients, enzymes, regulatory factors and transport molecules are present in uterine secretions. Enzymes include lysozyme, cathepsins B, D and E, aminoacylpeptidase, plasminogen activator, glucose phosphate isomerase, N-acetylglucosaminidase, hyaluronidase, oxytocinase, acid phosphatase (uteroferrin) and a number of glycosidases in pig uterine secretions. Glucose, fructose, riboflavin, ascorbic acid, sodium, potassium, calcium, amino acids, retinol, retinoic acid, prostaglandins and an extensive array of free and conjugated steroids are also found in uterine luminal fluid. Amounts of each of these components of uterine fluids are affected by day of the estrous cycle and stage of pregnancy. In general, uterine secretory activity is greatest when the uterus is under the influence of progesterone. However, estrogens can stimulate release of progesterone-induced proteins from secretory granules, as well as synthesis and secretion of estrogen-induced proteins. Events induced by the conceptus which result in release of endometrial secretory products and transport of substrate into the uterine lumen have been studied extensively in pigs (see 14,102).

Pig blastocysts begin to produce estrogens (40,45,49) and catecholestrogens (85) on Days 10.5-11 when they reach about 10mm diameter. These estrogens may act directly or indirectly, following conversion to catecholestrogens, to cause vasodilation of arterioles, increase uterine blood flow, stimulate uterine growth and endometrial secretory activity, stimulate uterine production of prostaglandins, induce an increase in endometrial receptors for prolactin and possibly alter effects of cholinergic and adrenergic agents on the uterine endometrium and myometrium (see 46).

Secretory vesicles accumulate in endometrial gland epithelium up to Days 10.5 to 12 of gestation and, in response to estrogens secreted by conceptuses, release their contents into the uterine lumen. This results in a marked increase in total protein, uteroferrin, protease inhibitors, PGF, PGE and calcium in uterine fluid. These changes can be induced in cyclic gilts within 12 to 24 h following administration of 5 mg estradiol valerate on Day 11. In pregnant gilts, there is an increase in calcium on Days 11-12, then total protein, PGF and PGE increase by Day 12-14, followed by an increase in sodium, potassium, and selected amino acids. Alanine, glycine, serine, tyrosine, arginine, histidine, isoleucine, leucine, lysine, methionine, phenylalanine, tryptophane and valine are higher in uterine flushings from pregnant than cyclic gilts (118). Glucose accumulates in uterine lumen after Day 12, but only in pregnant pigs, following the decrease in intraluminal calcium after Day 12. In cyclic gilts there are no significant changes in the composition of uterine fluid until after Day 14. Associated with the protracted decrease in calcium in cyclic gilts between Days 12 and 18 there is some increase in sodium and potassium, but no increase in glucose in uterine fluid. Selected androgens and progestins also increase in uterine flushing of pregnant gilts between Days 9 and 15 after onset of estrus (119). These include pregnenolone, progesterone, testosterone and dehydroepiandrosterone (DHEA) which can be converted to free estrogens by pig conceptuses. Concentrations of DHEA, for example, are about 40-fold higher in uterine flushings of pregnant gilts.

Pig endometrium and uterine secretions also contain β-endorphin (76) and methionine-enkephaline (77); however, their function(s) is not known. There is also an increase in the turnover of norepinephrine and dopamine, as well as an increase in cAMP and cGMP in endometrium of pregnant pigs in early pregnancy (129). These results suggest interactions between the conceptus and endometrium which change concentrations of cyclic nucleotides, catecholamines and opiods which may, in turn, affect uterine and conceptus functions during pregnancy. Proteins secreted by endometrial epithelium of sheep during early gestation have received limited attention. Total protein and activities of the enzymes succinic dehydrogenase, glutamic-oxaloacetic transaminase, acid phosphatase, alkaline phosphatase, glucose-6-phosphatase, beta-glucuronidase and glycogen phosphorylase are highest in uterine flushings from diestrus ewes and ovariectomized ewes treated with progesterone (see 6,90). Also, patterns of endometrial secretory proteins can be modified by injection of progesterone, transfer of an asynchronous conceptus into the uterine lumen or exposure of the endometrium to ovine conceptus secretory proteins or oTP-1 (7).

In addition to their roles as nutrients, enzymes and transport proteins, some secretory proteins have regulatory roles, e.g., regulation of the maternal immune system to allow survival of the conceptus allograft. Uterine secretions of the cow, sheep and pig contain proteins that inhibit the ability of mitogens to stimulate proliferation of lymphocytes in vitro. In addition, skin allografts placed into the uterine lumen are protected from rejection in ewes which have been ovariectomized and injected with progesterone for 30 days; the time required to stimulate secretion of two proteins (Mr = 57 and 59k) and referred to a ovine uterine milk proteins (oUTMP)(59). The endometrium and conceptuses of sheep, cows and pigs also secrete a high molecular weight glycoprotein which has immunosuppressive activity in vitro (91). The mechanism by which these presumed immunosuppressive proteins block a maternal cytotoxic attack on the conceptus is not known, but they could: (1) provide an immunoneutral zone surrounding the conceptus to prevent recognition of conceptus antigens by maternal lymphocytes; (2) suppress cloning of maternal lymphocytes and preventing development of significant antibody titers to conceptus antigens or (3) induce the maternal system to produce blocking antibodies to conceptus antigens to prevent their recognition by cytotoxic cells of the maternal immune system.

In pigs, uterine secretory activity is greatest between Days 12 and 16 and Days 35 and 75 of gestation when the progesterone:estrogen ratio is greatest. However, uterine secretory activity is also enhanced by prolactin (131) and prolactin receptors are highest (Days 35 to 75) when uterine secretory activity (33) and transport of nutrients into the fetal fluids (12) are greatest. In sheep, induction of secretion of oUTMP by progesterone requires about 30 days (84). In pregnant ewes the major increase in uterine secretory occurs after 90 days of gestation and is temporally associated with increased production of ovine placental lactogen (oPL) and increasing concentrations of progesterone in maternal plasma. It has been suggested (see 84) that oPL and/or prolactin, as well as estrogen, are necessary for induction of progesterone receptors and, in turn, induction of uterine secretory activity in ewes by progesterone. In sheep and pigs, placental lactogen (sheep) and/or prolactin, as well as estrogens may affect secretory function by regulating progesterone receptors in endometrial epithelium.

Uteroferrin, A Hematopoietic Growth Factor

The most extensively studied protein in uterine secretions of domestic animals is uteroferrin (UF). UF is a progesterone-induced glycoprotein secreted by the glandular epithelium of pig endometrium. UF has a Mr of about 35,000, a pI of about 9.7, acid phosphatase enzymatic activity and 2 molecules of iron per molecule of UF. The major role of UF has been presumed to be transport of iron from the uterine endometrium to the conceptus (103); however, UF has recently been shown to be a hematopoietic growth factor (44). The oligosaccharide chain of UF is of the high mannose type which may target UF to reticuloendothelial cells of the fetal liver; the major hematopoietic organ. Localization of UF in bone marrow and spleen has not been studied, but UF is also taken up by the yolk sac during early pregnancy (28). Iron from UF may be released to ferritin and transferred to erythroblasts by a process called ropheocytosis for synthesis of hemoglobin. Transcriptional activity of the UF gene is low, but distinct between Days 10 and 15 of pregnancy, declines to undetectable levels between Days 16 and 30 and then increases to maximal levels between Days 40 and term (115 days)(109). However, translation of mRNA for UF decreases after Day 60 of pregnancy in pigs; factors inhibiting translation of UF mRNA are not known. Two known inhibitors of tissue production of hematopoietic growth factors are lactoferrin (25) and a polypeptide (Mr 2,000) from bone marrow and liver of fetal calves at 6 to 7 months of gestation (58).

UF exists as the purple Mr 35,000 monomer and a rose-colored heterodimer (Rose) when bound to one of three UF-associated proteins (92). The UF-associated proteins have high amino acid sequence homology with serine protease inhibitors; however, the UF-associated proteins are not known to inhibit proteases (78). Both UF and Rose have colony forming unit (CFU) and burst forming unit (BFU) activities for erythroid (CFU-E) cells, as well as CFU-granulocyte-monocyte/macrophage (CFU-GM) and CFU-granulocyte-erythroid-monocyte/macrophage-megakaryocyte (CFU-GEMM) activities for myeloid cells when added to cultures of non-adherent hematopoietic stem cells from human bone marrow or neonatal piglet bone marrow, liver and spleen (44). oUTMP have Mr of 57,000 and 59,000 (10) and, like UF, high mannose carbohydrate chains, CFU-E, CFU-GM and CFU-GEMM hematopoietic growth factor activities (F.W. Bazer, D. Worthington-White, M.F.V. Fliss and S. Gross, unpublished results). oUTMP have high amino acid sequence homology with members of the serine protease inhibitor family (67). Crude bovine uterine secretions also have CFU-E, CFU-GM and CFU-GEMM hematopoietic growth factor activities (F.W. Bazer, D. Worthington-White, M.F.V. Fliss and S. Gross, unpublished results).

Human placenta also contains a UF-like protein referred to as tartrate resistant Type 5 acid phosphatase which has hematopoietic growth factor activity (F.W. Bazer, D. Worthington-White, M.A. Davis and S. Gross, unpublished results) and approximately 82% amino acid sequence homology with porcine UF (70, 113). Type 5 tartrate resistant acid phosphatases are also present in normal spleens of cattle, pigs and rats, diseased spleens of patients with hairy cell leukemia and Gaucher's disease, as well as patients with infectious mononucleosis, Pagets disease and osteoporosis (see 69). Collectively, these results suggest that uterine and/or placental tissues produce unique hematopoietic growth factors that may affect hematopoietic stem cells more primitive than those affected by E-CSF, GM-CSF and possibly interleukin-3 (multi-CSF).

Uterine epithelium of mice secrete monocyte/macrophage colony stimulating factor (CSF-1 or M-CSF) in response to ovarian steroids and values in the pregnant uterus are 1000-fold higher than during the estrous cycle (9). There is a corresponding increase in mRNA for CSF-1 in pregnant mouse uteri (99) indicating local synthesis of CSF-1 by mouse uterine endometrium.

Immunotrophism

Leukocytes are attracted to endometrial stroma during early pregnancy and, in sheep and pigs, localize beneath the basement membrane adjacent to developing conceptuses (71,75). Natural Killer cells (CD45R$^+$) are specifically recruited to endometrial stroma by pig and mouse conceptuses (32) and are the major granulated lymphocytes in endometrial epithelium and stroma of cyclic ewes (75). These cells appear to be more active, more abundant and limited to endometrial stroma of pregnant ewes until days 30 to 50 of pregnancy after which time they disappeared (56); an event temporally associated with the end of the second period of secretion of immunoreactive oTP-1 and the latter stages of placental development (98). Lymphocytes secrete interleukins (IL) 2,3,4,5 and 6, as well as gamma interferon and macrophages secrete IL-1 and IL-6, as well as GM-CSF, G-CSF, M-CSF, tumor necrosis factor (TNF), transforming growth factor-β (TGF-β), platelet derived growth factor (PDGF) and IFNα (95). These lymphokines and cytokines may stimulate conceptus development.

According to the theory of immunotrophism (127), lymphokines and cytokines secreted by leukocytes stimulate development of the trophectoderm. Trophectoderm then secretes steroid and protein paracrine hormones necessary for the establishment and maintenance of pregnancy, as well as transport nutrients and gases essential for survival of the conceptus.

Placental cells from mice have receptors for M-CSF and increase their rate of proliferation and phagocytic activity in response to both M-CSF and GM-CSF (127). Furthermore, DBA/2J female mice mated to CBA males have high rates of resorptions of conceptuses (24 of 51 conceptuses), small placentae (95 $\pm$ 16 mg) and low fetal weights (118 $\pm$ 20 mg)(127). However, DBA/2J females injected with 400 units GM-CSF/day have few conceptus resorptions (4 of 44), heavier placentae (138 $\pm$ 11 mg) and larger fetuses (211 $\pm$ 29 mg). This suggests a direct effect of CSF-1 on fetal/placental development in mice. UF and oUTMP, because of their GM-CSF and GEMM-CSF activities, may also stimulate proliferation of trophectoderm of pigs and sheep, as well as secretion of steroids and proteins by that tissue. Alternatively, UF and oUTMP may act in an additive or synergistic manner with lymphokines or cytokines, such as M-CSF from uterine epithelium, to stimulate proliferation and function of trophectodermal cells. In support of this hypothesis, passive immunization of pregnant pigs with antiserum to UF results in reduced placental length and weight at Day 60 of gestation (27).

Plasminogen Activator

Plasminogen activator of both the tissue (tPA) and urokinase (uPA) type are present in uterine secretions of pigs and may be involved in tissue remodelling, e.g., trophoblast outgrowth, implantation and uterine development, including angiogenesis (see 14, 102). The PA's are specific serine proteases which cleave the inactive zymogen plasminogen to the active plasmin. Progesterone-induced inhibitors of plasmin and possibly tPA and uPA are present in uterine secretions of pigs. These protease inhibitors may prevent invasive implantation of pig blastocysts, as is the case for PA from trophectoderm of rodent blastocysts. Pig blastocysts are invasive when transferred to ectopic sites, but not in the uterine lumen where protease inhibitors secreted by the endometrial surface epithelium are adsorbed to the trophectoderm. This may allow PA to affect remodelling of conceptus tissues, but prevent their invasive effects on uterine endometrium. Protease inhibitors may also protect secreted proteins, e.g., uteroferrin, from degradation in the uterine lumen or during transplacental transport into the fetal-placental circulation.

Growth Factors Secreted by the Endometrium

Growth factors known to be present in uterine tissue or uterine fluid (see 24,110,112) include insulin-like growth factor (IGF)-I (rat,pig), IGF-II (pig), Transforming Growth Factors α and β (TGFα and TGFβ, rat), acidic (α) and basic (β) Fibroblast Growth Factor (pig and human), Epidermal Growth Factor (EGF, mouse and rat), estromedins (now known to be IGF-1, rat and sheep) and uterine luminal fluid mitogens (ULFM, pig, 114). Growth factors are also produced by fetal-placental tissues (see 52). The presence of abundant mRNAs for IGF-I and IGF-II in uterine endometrium suggests autocrine and/or paracrine regulation of conceptus development by such factors (110,112).

What are the roles of growth factors secreted by the uterus? Are specific growth factors responsible for initiation of morphological development of conceptuses from spherical to tubular to filamentous forms and initiation of events leading to the secretion of steroids and/or proteins responsible for maternal recognition of pregnancy? Just prior to initiation of estrogen secretion and morphological transition from spherical, to tubular to filamentous forms, there is mesodermal outgrowth from the embryonic disc of pig conceptuses. It is during this period, i.e., Days 10 to 12 of pregnancy, that IGF-I is highest in uterine secretions of both cyclic and pregnant pigs. Furthermore, conceptuses of prolific Chinese Meishan pigs develop more rapidly (17), secrete more estrogens (18) and are exposed to higher amounts of IGF-I in uterine secretions than for less prolific Large White pigs (111). Secretion of significant amounts of IFNα-like proteins by pig conceptuses does not begin until Days 13 to 14 or well after mesodermal outgrowth is established. The growth factor associated with inducing mesoderm in amphibians is βFGF (72) and both αFGF and βFGF stimulate proliferation of mesoderm-derived cells (see 24). Fibroblast growth factors are believed to be present in pig endometrium and uterine secretions (24), but temporal associations between secretion of FGF, morphological changes in conceptuses and initiation of secretion of estrogens by pig conceptuses have not been established.

Initiation of secretion of oTP-1 occurs between Days 8 and 10 of pregnancy in sheep, but the most dramatic increase is between Days 10 and 14 when sheep conceptuses change from spherical, to tubular to filamentous organisms (7). On Day 13, changes in conceptus morphology are great and correlated with variation in total recoverable oTP-1 in uterine flushings: spherical conceptuses, 312 ng oTP-1; tubular conceptuses, 1380 ng oTP-1 and filamentous conceptuses, 4,455 ng oTP-1 (93). Results are not available to indicate which growth factors are present in uterine secretions of sheep or how they may affect conceptus development. However, co-culture of sheep endometrium and conceptuses recovered on Day 16 of pregnancy results in a two- to three-fold increase in secretion of oTP-1 into the culture medium which suggests that endometrial factors influence secretion of oTP-1 (8).

The rate of development of bovine conceptuses can be accelerated by injecting cows with exogenous progesterone (100 mg/day) on Days 1-4 after estrus (47). On Day 14, conceptuses from control cows averaged 3.8 ± 1.9 mm compared to 37.3 ± 14.9 mm in length for those from progesterone-treated cows. Bovine trophoblast protein-1 (bTP-1) was secreted by treated conceptuses which had an accelerated rate of development, but not control conceptuses. bTP-1, like oTP-1, is an interferon-like protein which, through its antiluteolytic effects, is responsible for maternal recognition of pregnancy in cattle.

Garrett et al. (47) were unable to detect qualitative effects of progesterone-treatment on proteins secreted by the endometrium following 2D-PAGE and flourography; however, proteins with Mr of 26,000 to 30,000 (pI values of 4.2-5.5) appeared in greater amounts on Day 5, while proteins with Mr of 21,000 (pI values of 6.3) and Mr of 22,000 to 26,000 (pI values of 7.9 to 8.9) appeared to be amplified on Day 14. Functional roles for those proteins have not been established. However, results of this study indicate that rate of conceptus development can be accelerated in progesterone-treated cattle. This model may be especially useful for examining interactions between the conceptus and endometrium that affect rate of morphological development of conceptuses and initiation of secretion of bTP-1.

Acknowledgements

Research from the University of Florida reported in this paper has been supported by National Institutes of Health Grant HD 10436 and U.S. Department of Agriculture Grant 86-CRCR-1-2106 and is published as University of Florida Agricultural Experiment Station Journal Series No. 18674. I wish to thank Drs. Rosalia C.M. Simmen and Frank A. Simmen, as well as Dr. Mark Mirando, Mr. Jacob P. Harney and Mr. Troy L. Ott for reviewing and contributing to the preparation of this paper and Dr. Samuel Gross, Diana Worthington-White and Filomema Fliss for collaborative work on hematopoietic growth factor activities of uteroferrin.

References

1. Acker, G., Braquet, P. and Mencia-Huerta, J.M. Role of platelet-activating factor (PAF) in the initiation of the decidual reaction in the rat. J. Reprod. Fertil. 85:623 (1989).
2. Acker, G., Hecquet, F., Etienne, A., Braquet, P., and Mencia-Huerta, J.M. Role of platelet-activating factor (PAF) in the ovoimplantation in the rat: effect of the specific PAF-acether antagonist, BN52021. Prostaglandins 35:233 (1988).
3. Adams, K.L., Bazer, F.W. and Roberts, R.M. Progesterone-induced secretion of a retinol-binding protein in the pig uterus. J. Reprod. Fertil. 62:39 (1981).
4. Albertini, D.F., Overstrom, E.W. and Ebert, K.M. Changes in the organization of the actin cytoskeleton during preimplantation development of the pig embryo. Biol. Reprod. 37:441 (1987).
5. Amatruda, T.T. and Koeffler, H.P. Retinoids and cells of the hematopoietic system. in: "Retinoids and Cell Differentiation", M.I. Sherman, ed., CRC Press, Boca Raton (1986).
6. Ashworth, C.J. 1985. Maternal factors affecting early pregnancy in sheep. Doctoral Thesis. University of Edinburgh, Edinburgh, Scotland.
7. Ashworth, C.J. and Bazer, F.W. Changes in ovine conceptus and endometrial function following synchronous embryo transfer and administration of progesterone. Biol. Reprod. 40:425 (1989).
8. Ashworth, C.J. and Bazer, F.W. Interrelationships of proteins secreted by the ovine conceptus and endometrium during the periattachment period. Anim. Reprod. Sci. 20:117 (1989).
9. Bartocci A., Pollard J.W., Stanley E.R. Regulation of colony stimulating factor during pregnancy. J. Exp. Med. 164:956 (1986).
10. Bazer, F.W. Vitamins in reproduction. in: "Proceedings of the Florida Nutrition Conference", St. Petersburg Beach, (1982).
11. Bazer, F.W., Roberts, R.M., Basha, S.M.M., Zavy, M.T., Caton, D. and Barron, D.H. Study of ovine uterine secretions obtained from unilaterally pregnant ewes. J. Anim. Sci. 49:1522 (1979).
12. Bazer, F.W., Goldstein, M.H. and Barron, D.H. Water and electrolyte transport by pig chorioallantois. in: "Fertilization and Embryonic Development In Vitro", J.D. Biggers and W.A. Sadler, eds., Plenum Publishing Corp. New York (1981).

13. Bazer, F.W. and First, N.L. Pregnancy and parturition. J. Anim. Sci. 57, Suppl. 2: 425 (1983).
14. Bazer, F.W. and Roberts, R.M. Biochemical aspects of conceptus-endometrial interactions. J. Exp. Zool. 228:373 (1984).
15. Bazer, F.W., Geisert, R.D., Thatcher, W.W. and Roberts, R.M. Endocrine vs exocrine secretion of $PGF_{2\alpha}$ in the control of pregnancy in swine. in: "Prostaglandins in Animal Reproduction II", L.E. Edqvist and H. Kindahl, eds. Elsevier Science Publishers, Amsterdam (1982).
16. Bazer, F.W., Vallet, J.L., Roberts, R.M., Sharp, D.C. and Thatcher, W.W. Role of conceptus secretory products in establishment of pregnancy. J. Reprod. Fert. 76:841 (1986).
17. Bazer, F.W., Thatcher, W.W., Martinat-Botte, F. and Terqui, M. Conceptus development in Large White and prolific Meishan pigs. J. Reprod. Fertil. 84:37 (1988).
18. Bazer, F.W., Thatcher, W.W., Martinat-Botte, F. and Terqui, M. 1987. Conceptus and uterine development in Large White and prolific Chinese Meishan gilts. J. Anim. Sci. 65, Suppl. 1:381 (1987).
19. Bazer, F.W., Vallet, J.L., Harney, J.P., Gross, T.S. and Thatcher, W.W. Comparative aspects of maternal recognition of pregnancy between sheep and pigs. J. Reprod. Fert. Suppl. 37, 85 (1989).
20. Beers, S., Mirando, M.A., Pontzer, C.H., Harney, J.P., Torres, B.A., Johnson, H.M. and Bazer, F.W. Influence of the endometrium, protease inhibitors and freezing on antiviral activity of proteins secreted by pig conceptuses. J. Reprod. Fertil. 88:205 (1990).
21. Blalock, J.E. and Gifford, G.E. Suppression of interferon production by vitamin A. J. Gen. Virol. 32:143 (1976).
22. Blalock, J.E. and Gifford, G.E. Retinoic acid (vitamin A acid) induced transcriptional control of interferon production. Proc. Natl. Acad. Sci. USA 74:5382 (1977).
23. Bramley, T.A. and Menzies, G.S. Receptor for lactogenic hormones in the porcine corpus luteum: properties and luteal phase concentrations. J. Endocrinol. 113:355 (1987).
24. Brigstock, D.R., Heap, R.B. and Brown, K.D. Polypeptide growth factors in uterine tissues and secretions. J. Reprod. Fertil. 85:747 (1989).
25. Broxmeyer, H.E., Smithyman, A., Eger, R.R., Meyers, P.A. and de Sousa, M. Identification of lactoferrin as the granulocyte-derived inhibitor of colony-stimulating activity production. J. Exp. Med. 148:1052 (1978).
26. Charpigny, G., Reinaud, P., Huet, J.C., Guillomot, M., Charlier, M., Pernallet, J.C. and Martal, J. High homology between trophoblastic protein (trophoblastin) isolated from ovine embryo and α-interferons. Fed. Europ. Biochem. Soc. 228:12 (1988).
27. Chen, T.T. and Bazer, F.W. Effects of antiserum to porcine fraction IV uterine protein on the conceptus. J. Anim. Sci. 37: 304 (1973).
28. Chen, T.T., Bazer, F.W., Gebhardt, B. & Roberts, R.M. Uterine secretion in mammals: Synthesis and placental transport of a purple acid phosphatase in pigs. Biol. Reprod. 13, 304 (1975).
29. Chiocca, E.A., Davies, P.J.A. and Stein, J.P. Regulation of tissue transglutaminase gene expression as a molecular model for retinoid effects on proliferation and differentiation. J. Cell Biochem. 39:293 (1989).
30. Cross, J.C. and Roberts, R.M. Porcine conceptuses secrete an interferon during the preattachment period of early pregnancy. Biol. Reprod. 40: 1109 (1989).
31. Croy, B.A., Wood, W. and King G.J. Evaluation of intrauterine immune suppression during pregnancy in a species with epitheliochorial placentation. J. Immunol. 139:1088 (1987).
32. Croy, B.A., Waterfield, A., Wood, W. and King, G.J. Normal murine and porcine embryos recruit NK cells to the uterus. Cell. Immunol. 115:471 (1988).
33. Dehoff, M., Bazer, F.W. and Collier, R.J. Ontogeny of prolactin receptors in porcine uterine endometrium during pregnancy. Proc. 4th Int. Prolactin Congr., Quebec p95 (1984)

34. Dimitrov, N.V., Meyer, C.J., Strander, H., Einhorn, S. and Cantell, K. Interferon as a modifier of estrogen receptors. Annals Clin. Lab. Sci. 14:32 (1984).

35. Ellinwood, W.E., Nett, T.M. and Niswender, G.D. Maintenance of the corpus luteum of early pregnancy in the ewe. I. Luteotropic properies of embryonic homogenates. Biol. Reprod. 21: 281 (1979).

36. Fairclough, R.J., Moore, L.G., Peterson, A.J. and Watkins, W.B. Effect of oxytocin on plasma concentrations of 13, 14-dihydro-15-keto prostaglandin F and the oxytocin associated neurophysin during the estrous cycle and early pregnancy in the ewe. Biol. Reprod. 31:36 (1984).

37. Faltynek, C.R., McCandless, S. and Baglioni, C. Treatment of lymphoblastoid cells with interferon decreases insulin binding. J. Cell Physiol. 121:437 (1984).

38. Fincher, K.B, Bazer, F.W., Hansen, P.J., Thatcher, W.W. and Roberts, R.M. Proteins secreted by the sheep conceptus suppress induction of uterine prostaglandin $F_{2\alpha}$ release by oestradiol and oxytocin. J. Reprod. Fert., 76:425 (1986).

39. Findlay, J.K., Clarke, I.J., Swaney, J., Colvin, N. and Doughton, B. Oestrogen receptors and protein synthesis in caruncular and intercaruncular endometrium of sheep before implantation. J. Reprod. Fertil. 64:329 (1982).

40. Fischer, H.E., Bazer, F.W. and Fields, M.J. Steroid metabolism by endometrial and conceptus tissues during early pregnancy and pseudopregnancy in gilts. J. Reprod. Fert. 75:69 (1985).

41. Flint, A.P.F. and Sheldrick, E.L. Ovarian oxytocin and maternal recognition of pregnancy. J. Reprod. Fert., 76:831 (1986).

42. Flint, A.P.F., Leat, W.M.R., Sheldrick, E.L. and Stewart, H.J. Stimulation of phosphoinositide hydrolysis by oxytocin and the mechanism by which oxytocin controls prostaglandin synthesis in the ovine endometrium. Biochem. J. 237:797 (1986).

43. Flechon, J.E., Guillomot, M., Charlier, M., Flechon,B. and Martal, J. Experimental studies on the elongation of the ewe blastocyst. Reprod. Nutr. Develop. 26:1017 (1986).

44. Fliss, M.F.V., Worthington-White,E., Gross, S. and Bazer, F.W. Uteroferrin and rose proteins from pig endometrium are hematopoietic growth factors. Biol. Reprod. 40, Suppl. 1:112 (1989).

45. Ford, S.P., Christenson, R.K. and Ford, J.J. Uterine blood flow and uterine arterial, venous and lumenal concentrations of oestrogens on days 11, 13 and 15 after oestrus in pregnant and nonpregnant sows. J. Reprod. Fert. 64:185 (1982).

46. Ford, S.P. Factors controlling uterine blood flow during estrus and early pregnancy. in: "The Uterine Circulation", C. Rosenfeld, ed., Perinatology Press, Ithaca (1989).

47. Garrett, J.E., Geisert, R.D., Zavy, M.T. and Morgan, G.L. Evidence for maternal regulation of early conceptus growth and development in the bovine. J. Reprod. Fertil. 84:437 (1988).

48. Garverick, H.A., Polge, C. and Flint, A.P.F. Oestradiol administration raises luteal LH receptor levels in intact and hysterectomized pigs. J. Reprod. Fertil. 66:371 (1982).

49. Geisert, R.D., Renegar, R.H., Thatcher, W.W., Roberts, R.M. and Bazer, F.W. Establishment of pregnancy in the pig. I. Interrelationships between preimplantation development of the pig blastocyst and uterine endometrial secretions. Biol. Reprod. 27:925 (1982).

50. Geisert,R.D., Brookbank, J.W., Roberts, R.M. and Bazer, F.W. Establishment of pregnancy in the pig. II. Cellular remodelling of porcine blastocysts during elongation on day 12 of pregnancy. Biol. Reprod. 27:941 (1982).

51. Geisert, R.D., Zavy, M.T., Wettemann, R.P. and Biggers, B.G. Length of pseudopregnancy and pattern of uterine protein release as influenced by time and duration of estrogen administration in the pig. J. Reprod. Fertil. 39: 163 (1987).

52. Gluckman, P.D. The regulation of fetal growth. in: "Control and Manipulation of Fetal Growth". P.J.Buttery, H.B. Haynes and D.B. Lindsay, eds., Butterworths, London (1986).

53. Godkin, J.D., Bazer, F.W., Moffat, R.J., Sessions, F. and Roberts, R.M. Purification and properties of a major, low molecular weight protein released by the trophoblast of sheep blastocysts at Day 13-21. J. Reprod. Fert. 65:141 (1982).

54. Godkin, J.D., Bazer, F.W., Lewis, G.S., Geisert, R.D. and Roberts, R.M. Synthesis and release of polypeptides by pig conceptuses during the period of blastocyst elongation and attachment. Biol. Reprod. 27:977 (1982).

55. Godkin, J.D., Bazer, F.W. and Roberts, R.M. Ovine trophoblast protein-1, an early secreted blastocyst protein, binds specifically to uterine endometrium and affects protein synthesis. Endocrinology 114:120 (1984).

56. Gogolin-Ewens, K. Personal communication. (1988)

57. Gross, T.S., Lacroix, M.C., Bazer, F.W., Thatcher, W.W. and Harney, J.P. Prostaglandin secretion by perifused porcine endometrium: further evidence for an endocrine versus exocrine secretion of prostaglandins. Prostaglandins 35:327 (1988).

58. Guigon, M. and Wdzieczak-Bakala, J. Hemopoietic stem cell regulators in fetal liver. in: "Fetal Liver Transplantation", eds. Alan R. Liss, Inc., Philadelphia (1985).

59. Hansen, P.J., Bazer, F.W. and Segerson, E.C. Skin graft survival in the uterine lumen of ewes treated with progesterone. Am. J. Reprod. Immunol. Microbiol. 12:48 (1986).

60. Harney, J.P. and Bazer, F.W. Effect of porcine conceptus secretory proteins on inter-estrous interval and uterine secretion of prostaglandins. Biol. Reprod. 41:277 (1989).

61. Harney, J.P. and Mirando, M.A. Retinol-binding protein: A major secretory product of the pig conceptus. Biol. Reprod. 40 (Suppl. 1):131 (1989).

62. Harney, J.P., Mirando, M.A. and Bazer, F.W. Characterization of antiviral activity of proteins secreted by the pig conceptus. J. Anim. Sci. 67, Suppl.1:403 (1989).

63. Harper, M.J.K. Platelet-activating factor: A paracrine factor in preimplantation stages of reproduction. Biol. Reprod. 40:907 (1989).

64. Hixon, J.E. and Flint, A.P.F. Effects of a luteolytic dose of oestradiol benzoate on uterine oxytocin receptor concentrations, phosphoinositide turnover and prostaglandin F-2α secretion in sheep. J. Reprod. Fertil. 79:457 (1987).

65. Hooper, S.B., Watkins, W.B. and Thorburn, G.D. Oxytocin, oxytocin associated neurophysin, and prostaglandin $F_{2\alpha}$ concentrations in the utero-ovarian vein of pregnant and nonpregnant sheep. Endocrinology 119:2590 (1986).

66. Imakawa, K., Anthony, R.V., Kazemi, M., Maroti, K.R., Polites, H.G. and Roberts, R.M. Interferon-like sequence of ovine trophoblast protein secreted by embryonic trophec-toderm. Nature, Lond. 330:377 (1987).

67. Ing, N.H. "The Uterine Milk Proteins: Structure, Biosynthesis and Function". Doctoral Dissertation, University of Florida, Gainesville (1988).

68. Kauppila, A., Cantell, K., Janne, O., Kokko, E. and Vihko, R. Serum sex steroid and peptide hormone concentrations and endometrial estrogen and progesterone receptor levels during administration of human leukocyte interferon. Int. J. Cancer 29:291 (1982).

69. Ketcham, C.M., Baumbach, G.A., Bazer, F.W. and Roberts, R.M. The type 5 acid phosphatase from spleen of humans with hairy cell leukemia; purification, properties, immunological characterization and comparison with porcine uteroferrin. J. Biol. Chem. 260:5768 (1985).

70. Ketcham, C.M., Roberts, R.M., Simmen, R.C.M. and Nick, H.S. Molecular cloning of the type 5, iron-containing, tartrate-resistant acid phosphatase from human placenta. J. Biol. Chem. 264:557 (1989).

71. Keys, J.L. Structural changes in porcine uterine epithelium during the estrous cycle, early pregnancy and pseudopregnancy. Doctoral Dissertation. University of Guelph, Guelph (1987).

72. Kimelman, D., Abraham, J.A., Haaparanta, T., Palisi, T.M. and Kirschner, M.W. The presence of fibroblast growth factor in the frog egg: its role as a natural mesoderm inducer. Science 242:1053 (1988).

73. Kittok, R.J. and Britt, J.H. Corpus luteum function in ewes given estradiol during the estrous cycle or early pregnancy. J. Anim. Sci. 45:336 (1977).

74. Lacroix, M.C. and Kann, G. Discriminating analysis of in vitro prostaglandin release by myometrial and luminal sides of the ewe endometrium. Prostaglandins 25:853 (1983).

75. Lee, C.S., Gogolin-Ewens, K. and Brandon, M.R. Identification of a unique lymphocyte subpopulation in the sheep uterus. Immunology 63:157 (1988).

76. Li, W.I., Chen, C.L., Hansen, P.J. and Bazer, F.W. β-Endorphin in uterine secretions of pseudopregnant and ovariectomized, ovarian steroid-treated gilts. Endocrinology 121:1111 (1987).

77. Li, W.I. and Sung, L.C. Immunoreactive methionine-enkephalin in porcine reproductive tissues. Biol. Reprod. 40, Suppl. 1:78 (1989).

78. Malathy, P.V. and Imakawa, K. Uteroferrin-associated basic protein, a major progesterone-induced secretory protein of the porcine uterus, is a member of the serpin superfamily of protease inhibitors. Biol. Reprod. 40, Suppl. 1:114 (1989).

79. McCracken, J.A., Schramm, W. and Okulicz, W.C. Hormone receptor control of pulsatile secretion of $PGF_{2\alpha}$ from the ovine uterus during luteolysis and its abrogation in early pregnancy. in: "Prostaglandins in Animal Reproduction II", L. E. Edqvist and H. Kindahl, eds. Elsevier, Amsterdam (1984).

80. Milligan, S.R. and Finn, C.A. Failure to demonstrate platelet activating factor involvement in implantation in mice. J. Reprod. Fert. Abstract Series 2:29 (1988).

81. Mirando, M.A., Gross, T.S., Young, K.H. and Bazer, F.W. Reorientation of prostaglandin F(PGF) secretion by calcium ionophore, oestradiol and prolactin in perifused porcine endometrium. J. Reprod. Fertil. Abstract Series 1:58 (1988).

82. Mirando, M.A., Harney, J.P., Beetrs, S., Pontzer, C.H., Torres, B.A., Johnson, H.M. and Bazer, F.W. Onset of secretion of proteins with antiviral activity by pig conceptuses. J. Reprod. Fertil. 88:197 (1990).

83. Mirando, M.A., Ott, T.L., Vallet, J.L., Davis, M.A. and Bazer, F.W. Oxytocin-stimulated inositol phosphate turnover in endometrium of ewes is influenced by stage of the estrous cycle, pregnancy and intrauterine infusion of ovine conceptus secretory proteins. Biol. Reprod. 42:98 (1990).

84. Moffatt, R.J., Bazer, F.W., Hansen, P.J., Chun, P.W. and Roberts, R.M. Purification and immunocytochemical localization of the uterine milk proteins, the major progesterone-induced proteins in uterine secretions of sheep. Biol. Reprod. 36:419 (1987).

85. Mondschein, J.S., Hersey, R.M., Dey, S.K., Davis, D.L. and Weisz, J. Catecholestrogen formation by pig blastocysts during the preimplantation period: Biochemical characterization of estrogen-2/4-hydroxylase and correlation with aromatase activity. Endocrinology 117:2339 (1985).

86. Moor, R.M. and Rowson, L.E.A. The corpus luteum of the sheep: Effect of the removal of embryos on luteal function. J. Endocrinol. 34:497 (1966).

87. Moor, R.M. and Rowson, L.E.A. The corpus luteum of the sheep: Functional relationship between the embryo and the corpus luteum. J. Endocrinol. 34:233 (1966).

88. Morgan, G.L., Geisert, R.D., Zavy, M.T. and Fazleabas, A.T. Development and survival of pig blastocysts after oestrogen administration on Day 9 or Days 9 and 10 of pregnancy. J. Reprod. Fertil. 80:133 (1987).

89. Morton, H. EPF as a pregnancy protein. in: "Early pregnancy factor". F.Ellendorf and E. Koch, eds., Perinatology Press, Ithaca, (1985).

90. Murdoch, B.E. and O'Shea, T. Activity of enzymes in the mucousal tissues and rinsings of the reproductive tract of the naturally cyclic ewe. Aust. J. Biol. Sci. 31:345 (1978).

91. Murray, M.K., Segerson, E.C., Hansen, P.J., Bazer, F.W. and Roberts, R.M. Suppression of lymphocyte activation by a high molecular weight glycoprotein released from preimplantation ovine and porcine conceptuses. Am. J. Reprod. Immunol. Microbiol. 14:38 (1987).

92. Murray, M.K., Malathy, P.V., Bazer, F.W. and Roberts, R.M. Structural relationship, biosynthesis, and immunocytochemcial localization of uteroferrin-associated basic glycoproteins. J. Biol. Chem. 264:4143 (1989).

93. Nephew, K.P., McClure, K.E. Ott, T.L., Bazer, F.W. and Pope, W.F. Cumulative recognition of pregnancy by embryonic production of ovine trophoblastic protein-one. J. Anim. Sci.67, Suppl. 1:404 (1989).

94. Newton, G.R., Vallet, J.L., Hansen, P.J. and Bazer, F.W. Inhibition of lymphocyte proliferation by ovine trophoblast protein-1 and a high molecular weight glycoprotein

produced by preimplantation sheep conceptus. Am. J. Reprod. Immunol. Microbiol. 19:99 (1989).

95. Old, L.L. Tumor necrosis factor. Sci. Am. 258:59 (1988).
96. O'Neill, C. Embryo-derived platelet activating factor: a preimplantation embryo mediator of maternal recognition of pregnancy. Domestic Anim. Endocrinol. 4:69 (1987).
97. O'Neill, C., Collier, M., Ryan, J.P. and Spinks, R.N. Embryo-derived platelet-activating factor. J. Reprod. Fert. Suppl. 37:19 (1989).
98. Ott, T.L., Mirando, M.A., Davis, M.A., Fliss, M.F.V. and Bazer, F.W. Characterization of a second period of immunoreactive ovine trophoblast protein-one secretion in sheep. J. Anim. Sci. 67, Suppl. 1:370 (1989).
99. Pollard, J.W., Bartocci, A., Areci, R., Orlofsky, A., Ladner, M.B. and Stanley, E.R. Apparent role of the macrophage growth factor, CSF-1, in placental development. Nature, London 330:484 (1987).
100. Pontzer, C.H., Torres, B.Z., Vallet, J.L., Bazer, F. W. and Johnson, H.M. Antiviral activity of the pregnancy recognition hormone ovine trophoblast protein-1. Biochem. Biophys. Res. Commun. 152:801 (1988).
101. Pottathil, R., Chandrabose, K.A., Cuatrecasas, P. and Lang, D.J. Establishment of the interferon-mediated antiviral state: Role of fatty acid cyclooxygenase. Proc. Natl. Acad. Sci., USA 77:5437 (1980).
102. Roberts, R.M. and Bazer, F.W. The functions of uterine secretions. J. Reprod. Fertil. 82:875 (1988).
103. Roberts, R.M., Raub, T.J. and Bazer, F.W. Role of uteroferrin in transplacental iron transport in the pig. Fed. Proc. 45:2513 (1986).
104. Schindler, J. Retinoids, polyamines and differentiation. in: "Retinoids and Cell Differentiation", M.I. Sherman, ed., CRC Press, Boca Raton (1986).
105. Sheldrick, E.L. and Flint, A.P.F. Endocrine control of uterine oxytocin receptors in the ewe. J. Endocrinol. 106:249 (1985).
106. Shille, V.M., Karlbom, I., Einarsson, S., Larsson, K., Kindahl, H. and Edqvist, L.E. Concentrations of progesterone and 15-keto-13, 14-dihydroprostaglandin $F_{2\alpha}$ in peripheral plasma during the estrous cycle and early pregnancy in gilts. Zentbl. Vet. Med.A 26:169 (1979).
107. Short, R.V. Implantation and the maternal recognition of pregnancy, in: "Foetal Autonomy", Ciba Foundation Symposium. Churchill, London (1969).
108. Silvia, W.J., Ottobre, J.S. and Inskeep, E.K. Concentrations of prostaglandins E_2, $F_{2\alpha}$ and 6-keto-prostaglandin $F_{1\alpha}$ in the utero-ovarian venous plasma of nonpregnant and early pregnant ewes. Biol. Reprod. 30:936 (1984).
109. Simmen, R.C.M., Baumbach, G. and Roberts, R.M. Molecular cloning and temporal expression during pregnancy of the messenger ribonucleic acid encoding uteroferrin, a progesterone-induced uterine secretory protein. Mol. Endocrinol. 2:253 (1988).
110. Simmen, R.C.M. and Simmen, F.A. Regulation of uterine and conceptus secretory activity in the pig. J. Reprod. Fertil. Suppl. 40:279 (1990).
111. Simmen, R.C.M., Simmen, F.A., Ko, Y. and Bazer, F.W. Differential growth factor content of uterine luminal fluids from Large White and prolific Meishan pigs during the estrous cycle and early pregnancy. J. Anim. Sci. 67:1538 (1989).
112. Simmen, F.A., Simmen, R.C.M. and Bazer, F.W. Maternal growth factors as mediators of embryonic and neonatal growth. Biochem. Soc. Trans. 17:587 (1988).
113. Simmen, R.C.M., Srinivas, V. and Roberts, R.M. Complementary sequence, gene organization and production of messenger RNA for uteroferrin, a porcine uterine iron transport protein. DNA 8:543 (1989).
114. Simmen, R.C.M., Ko, Y., Liu, X.H., Wilde, M.H., Pope, W.F. and Simmen, F.A. A uterine cell mitogen distinct from epidermal growth factor in porcine uterine luminal fluids: characterization and partial purification. Biol. Reprod. 38:551 (1988).
115. Spinks, N.R. and O'Neill, C. Embryo-derived platelet-activating factor is essential for establishment of pregnancy in the mouse. Lancet 1:106 (1987).

116. Spinks, N.R. and O'Neill, C. Antagonists of embryo-derived platelet-activating factor prevent implantation in the mouse. J. Reprod. Fertil. 84:89 (1988).

117. Stewart, H.J., McCann, S.H.E., Barker, P.J., Lee, K.E., Lamming, G.E. and Flint,A.P.F. Interferon sequence homology and receptor binding activity of ovine trophoblast antiluteolytic protein. J. Endocrinol. 115, R13 (1987).

118. Stone, B.A. "Biochemical Aspects of Early Pregnancy", Doctoral Dissertation, University of Adelaide, Adelaide (1985).

119. Stone, B.A. and Seamark, R.F. Steroid hormones in uterine washings and in plasma of gilts between Days 9 and 15 after oestrus and between Days 9 and 15 after coitus. J. Reprod. Fertil. 75:209 (1985).

120. Taylor-Papadimitriou, J. and Rozengurt, E. Interferons as regulators of cell growth and differentiation. in: "Interferons: Their Impact In Biology and Medicine". J Taylor-Papadimitriou, ed. Oxford University Press, Oxford (1985).

121. Thatcher, W.W., Hansen, P.J., Gross, T.S., Helmer, S.D., Plante, C. and Bazer, F.W. Antiluteolytic effects of bovine trophoblast protein-1. J. Reprod. Fertil. Suppl. 37:91 (1989).

122. Thatcher, W.W., Knickerbocker, J.J., Bartol, F.F., Bazer, F.W., Roberts, R.M. and Drost, M. Maternal recognition of pregnancy in relation to survival of transferred embryos: endocrine aspects. Theriogenology 23:129 (1985).

123. Vallet, J.L., Bazer, F.W., Fliss, M.F. V. and Thatcher, W.W. Effect of ovine conceptus secretory proteins and purified ovine trophoblast protein-1 on interoestrous interval and plasma concentrations of prostaglandins F-2α and E and of 13, 14-dihydro-15-keto prostaglandin F-2α in cyclic ewes. J. Reprod. Fertil. 84:493 (1988).

124. Vallet, J.L., Gross, T.S., Fliss, M.F.V. and Bazer, F.W. Effects of pregnancy, oxytocin, ovine trophoblast protein-1 and their interactions on endometrial production of prostaglandin $F_{2\alpha}$ in vitro in perifusion chambers. Prostaglandins 38:113 (1989).

125. Vallet, J.L. and Bazer, F.W. The effect of ovine trophoblast protein-1, oestrogen and progesterone on oxytocin-induced phosphatidylinositol turnover in endometrium of sheep. J. Reprod. Fertil. 87: (In Press) (1989)

126. Waters, M.J., Oddy, V.H., McCloghry, C.E., Gluckman, P.D., Duplock, R., Owens, P.C. and Brinsmead, M.W. An examination of the proposed roles of placental lactogen in the ewe by means of antibody neutralization. J. Endocrinol. 106:377 (1985).

127. Wegmann, T.G. Maternal T cells promote placental growth and prevent spontaneous abortion. Immunol. Letters. 17:297 (1988).

128. Wilson, M.E., Lewis, G.S. and Bazer, F.W. Proteins of ovine blastocyst origin. Biol. Reprod. 20 (Suppl. 1): 101 (1979).

129. Young, K.H., Bazer, F.W., Simpkins, J.W. and Roberts, R.M. Effects of early pregnancy and acute 17β-estradiol administration on porcine uterine secretion, cyclic nucleotides and catecholamines. Endocrinology 120:254 (1987).

130. Young, K.H. Estrogens regulate porcine endometrial prolactin receptors. Biol. Reprod. 40, Suppl. 1:130 (1989).

131. Young, K.H., Kraeling, R.R. and Bazer, F.W. Effects of prolactin on conceptus survival and uterine secretory activity in pigs. J. Reprod. Fertil. 86:713 (1989).

132. Zarco, L., Stabenfeldt, G. H., Quirke, J.F., Kindahl, H.and Bradford, G.E. Release of prostaglandin F-2α and the timing of events associated with luteolysis in ewes with oestrous cycles of different lengths. J. Reprod. Fert. 83:517 (1988).

133. Zarco, L., Stabenfeldt, G.H., Basu, S., Bradford, G.E. and Kindahl, H. Modification of prostaglandin F-2α synthesis and release in the ewe during the initial establishment of pregnancy. J.Reprod.Fert. 83:527 (1988).

Questions

Dr. Bern: No one has done a systematic study of the types of hormones seen in uterine secretions. There must be some there, as well as growth factors. I wondered what information you have in this area?

Dr. Bazer: Unfortunately, there is a fairly limited amount of information that quite a few of the steroids, progestogens, androgens, estrogens, in the free unconjugated form are present there. There is some evidence for oxytocin being released into the uterine lumen of the pig, β-endorphin from David Chen's work is known to be there. The pig endometrium does not seen to produce prolactin nor does the placenta seem to produce placental lactogen. But what seems to happen is that the estrogen production by the pig conceptus is triphasic: day 10-12, 16-30, 75-term and what it does is modulate prolactin receptors on the endometrium. So we think that there it is really modulation of receptor numbers, even though the circulating level of Prolactin remains relatively constant. There is a GNRH-associated protein which David Chen has found in the pig endometrium. I'm not really sure anybody has looked for growth hormone, TSH, T3 or T4; I've not seen any data. Ken Polakowski has analyzed uterine secretions for insulin and could not detect any in pig uterine secretions.

Dr. Short: I was interested in how you visualized the effects of the water soluble hormones such as oxytocin?

Dr. Bazer: Well if it works through the classical system it would activate phospholipase c, which would give you inositol phosphate which would then go to IP_3 and so forth and activate the calcium-calmodulin kinase system and the diacyl glycerol would activate protein kinase C.

Dr. Short: Has anyone measured diacyl glycerol or protein kinase C in the pig or sheep endometrium?

Dr. Bazer: We have not measured either one of those. The thing we've measured showed that there was an increase in inositol phosphate turnover. So far as I'm aware no one has actually measured diacyl glycerol or protein kinase c directly in the sheep endometrium either. So it's really based on the one arm of the second messenger system that people have focused on.

Dr. Glasser: I was impressed with your two dimensional gels showing secretions. We have two-dimensional gels which looked a lot like that, and there are relatively few proteins in these gels. It looks like, qualitatively there aren't many proteins.

Dr. Bazer: Right, in the sheep that's true.

Dr. Carson: You mentioned something about membrane-associated protein which got released by the uterus. My first question is: are they released along with membrane fragments or proteolytic fragments? The second question is in regard to the vitamin A binding proteins, are they secreted with bound vitamin A or are they not?

Dr. Bazer: Well, if you look at the pig epithelium its sort of like a roe deer in delayed implantation from about day four or five in gestation, a lot of proteins are synthesized and packaged in the secretory vesicles in the pig epithelium, and with the pig estrogen and calcium there is just a huge dumping of all that protein. There are membrane-associated enzymes. We use this acyl aminopeptidase as an index of a membrane processing in both exocytosis and endocytosis. I believe the retinoid binding proteins are released with retinoids attached to them, because Cathy Adams measured vitamin A in uterine secretions and they followed these proteins out.

Dr. Leavitt: I have a question about the oxytocin receptors. According to some, progesterone down regulates after estrogen up regulation. Presumably that does not decrease sensitivity to oxytocin activity. You mentioned that you are testing oTP-1 as a conditional factor. How do you think the hormones work; is there a progesterone effect on the oviduct?

Dr. Bazer: If you take a cycling sheep and take the ovaries out and treat the animals with progesterone, initially you get an increase in oxytocin receptors after three or four days. After five days they start going down again and they go into what McCracken has referred to as a progesterone block and that lasts for about eleven days. If you give progesterone early you can shift it back toward estrous. That is, if you start progesterone prematurely. So it seems like there is an eleven day period where progesterone can do its thing. When it comes out of the block, whatever that means, then the oxytocin receptors come back up. I think estrogen facilitates that. In the sheep or cow, if we give a GnRH analogue, so that we can keep knocking the follicle back down into atresia we can keep the corpus luteum going as long as we keep giving GnRH every three days. So I think those two tie in together. I think on a progesterone background, estrogen helps to up regulate oxytocin receptors.

In terms of how oTP-1 acts, we don't know whether it is acting at the level of the genome or the cytoskeleton. I think that it is probably acting to block the synthesis of the receptor or its insertion into the membrane. Our bias is toward the synthesis, but that's only speculation at the moment. One of the properties of α-interferon, if you treat patients with tumors is that they cause tumor cells to become depleted of lactoferrin and transferrin receptors and cholera toxin receptors. So there is precedence for thinking that an interferon-like molecule could block receptor formation or recycling.

11

The Endocrine Function of the Rodent Placenta: Placental Lactogens

F. Talamantes, J. N. Southard, L. Ogren, and G. Thordarson
Department of Biology, Sinsheimer Laboratories
University of California
Santa Cruz, California 95064

Summary

Placental lactogens are prolactin and growth hormone-like hormones produced by the fetal placenta of a variety of mammalian species. Mouse placental lactogen-I (mPL-I), mouse placental lactogen-II (mPL-II) and hamster placental lactogen-II (haPL-II) have been purified and characterized at the protein and cDNA level. Mouse-PL-I is a single chain glycosylated polypeptide of 194 amino acid residues, containing 5 cysteine residues and 2 sites for N-linked glycosylation. Mouse-PL-II is a single chain polypeptide of 191 amino acid residues, containing 5 cysteine residues and no carbohydrate moieties. Hamster PL-II is also a single chain polypeptide of 191 amino acid residues, containing 5 cysteine residues and no carbohydrate moieties. By immunocytochemistry, mPL-II has been localized to the placental giant cells. Utilizing a homologous RIA, the concentration mPL-I has been found to be detected as early as day 6 of pregnancy with peak levels on day 10 of gestation. In contrast, circulating mPL-II is first detected on day 10 of pregnancy, and the hormone level increases until term. The maternal serum mPL-II concentration is regulated by the number of conceptuses, the genotype of the feto-placental unit, by the pituitary via growth hormone, the maternal nutritional status, ovaries and the decidua. An increase in the production rate of mPL-II appears to play a role in determining the gestational profile of the hormone but a change in half-life does not. Receptors for mPL-I and mPL-II have been characterized on ovarian and hepatic tissue from pregnant mice. Both haPL-II, mPL-I and mPL-II have been shown to have *in vitro* lactogenic activity in mouse mammary tissue.

Introduction

The mammalian placenta has been shown to be a very versatile endocrine organ. Numerous studies have demonstrated that the placenta is the site of synthesis and secretion of steroid, protein and polypeptide hormones (23,29). In general, the placental protein and polypeptide hormones have been shown to be structurally and functionally very comparable to protein and polypeptide hormones produced by the pituitary gland and hypothalamus. Thus, the placentae of several mammalian species produce: (a) a placental lactogen (PL), which shares properties with prolactin (PRL) and growth hormone (GH); (b) a chorionic gonadotropin (CG), which is similar to lutropin (LH); (c) a group of peptides derived from a pro-opiomelancortin-like molecule; and (d) a number of polypeptides that are very similar to the hypothalamic releasing and inhibiting hormones. The placenta of several species synthesize relaxin, which is also produced by the ovaries. In addition, the feral component of the rat (9, 10), mouse (18,19) and bovine (29) placenta produces molecules that have amino acid sequence homology to pituitary PRL. In this chapter, we will discuss the

Cellular Signals Controlling Uterine Function
Edited by L.A. Lavia, Plenum Press, New York

biochemical structure of mouse and hamster PL, regulation of secretion and function of mouse PL's.

Structure

Mouse placental lactogen-I is a glycoprotein composed of species that range in molecular weight from about 29K to 42K, as determined by SDS polyacrylamide gel electrophoresis (4). Most of the molecular weight heterogeneity between mPL-I species is due to differences in glycosylation. Sequence analysis of a cDNA for mPL-I suggests that it is synthesized as a 224-amino acid precursor and secreted as a 194-amino acid species (5). The predicted amino acid sequence includes two potential sites for asparagine-linked glycosylation and 5 cysteine (cys) residues. The odd number of cys residues in mPL-I is an unusual feature among PLs. The "extra" cys, cys 167, is thought to form a disulfide bond with cys 169, which in other members of the PRL-GH-PL family participates in the formation of the large disulfide loop structure that is characteristic of this family of hormones. Formation of disulfide bond between cys 167 and 169 is thought to prevent the formation of the large disulfide loop in mPL-I. The N-linked oligosaccharides of mPL-I are of the complex or hybrid type and contain sialic acid. Including the signal sequence, mPL-I shares 44% amino acid homology with mPL-II, 33% identity with mouse prolactin (mPRL) and 20% identity with mouse growth hormone (mGH).

Mouse PL-II is a single chain polypeptide having a molecular weight of 21, 812 (3,16). Sequence analysis of the cDNA indicates that the hormone is synthesized as a 222-amino acid precursor which is cleaved to yield a 191 amino acid mature mPL-II molecule. There are four cys residues. Although the position of the disulfide bonds has not been determined, they are predicted to occur between cys 51 and 166 and cys 183 and 191 by analogy to mPRL and mGH. Mouse PL-II exists as several charge isoforms with isoelectric points ranging from 7.0 to 6.6 (34). The amino acid sequence of mPL-II shows 51% sequence homology with mPRL and 31% sequence homology with mGH.

Sequence analysis of the cDNA for hamster placental lactogen-II (haPL-II) codes for 221 amino acid precursor protein which is cleaved to yield a 191 amino acid mature haPL-II protein (35,36). As is the case for mPL-II and rat placental lactogen-II (rPL-II), the mature haPL-II does not contain a consensus sequence for Asn-linked glycosylation (Asn-X-Ser\Thr). The most obvious structural difference between haPL-II and the other rodent PLs is the presence of an additional pair of cysteine (Cys) residues. The four Cys residues of haPL-II which correspond to those of mPL-II and rPL-II (at positions 51, 166,183 and 191) are conserved in all known members of the GH-PRL-PL family. In addition, haPL-II contains a pair of Cys residues not present in the other rodent PLs. These occur at residue 21 (Asn in mPL-II (and Tyr in rPL-II) and residue 42 (Trp in MPL-II and rPL-II). This unique pair of Cys residues may be responsible for the extreme tendency of haPL-II, compared to other members of the GH-PRL-PL family, to form disulfide-bonded hormone-serum protein complexes (37). Overall, haPL-II has essentially identical sequence homology to both mPL-II (70% identity) and rPL-II (68% identity). This homology is slightly less than between mPL-II and rPL-II (79% identity).

Sequence analysis of the cDNA for rPL-II indicates that the mature molecule consists of 191 amino acids (8). Unlike hPL which is 85% homologous to human growth hormone (hGH) at the amino acid level, rPL-II is much more closely related to the PRLs. Thus, rPL-II is 52% homologous to rat prolactin at the amino acid level, but only 34% related to rat growth hormone.

Secretion

Mouse PL-I is produced by cells of the chorioallantoic and choriovitelline placentas (14,31). This hormone has been localizes to the giant cells and basophilic cytotrophoblasts by immunohistochemical methods (14). The distribution of giant cells that contain mPL-II changes during pregnancy. At midpregnancy, mPL-II is present primarily in giant cells of the decidua capsularis and the basal zone. As pregnancy advances, giant cells of the labyrinth become mPL-II positive; those of the decidua capsularis and basal zone lose staining for mPL-II. By immunocytochemistry, rPL-II has also been localized to the placental giant cells (2).

Utilizing a homologous radioimmunoassay (RIA), mPL-I appears in maternal serum on day 6 of pregnancy. Its concentration remained low until day 8 and then increased to a very large peak on days 9 to 11 (maximum concentration @ 8 μg\ml). The mPL-I concentration declined after day 11, the hormone could be detected at low concentration in maternal serum until the end of pregnancy. On day 10 of gestation, the mPL-I concentration of the maternal serum was correlated with litter size (24).

On the other hand, mPL-II appears in the maternal circulation on day 9 of pregnancy, and its concentration increases until about day 14 (30). After day 14, the serum profile of mPL-II differs between mouse strains. In C3H mice, serum mPL-II concentration remains constant after day 14 (about 100 ng\ml); in the BALB\c and Swiss Webster strains, the mPL-II concentrations continues to increase after day 14 until term (>250 ng\ml) (30,33). Mouse PL-II is cleared very rapidly from the maternal circulation with biexponential kinetics; the half-life of the rapid phase is about 18 minutes (25). The clearance rate of mPL-I has not yet been determined.

Several factors that influence the concentration of mPL-II in the maternal circulation have been identified. They include litter size, the genotype of the feto-placental unit, the pituitary, the ovaries and the nutritional status of the mother. The maternal serum mPL-II concentration is positively correlated with the number of conceptuses (32). It is likely that this effect of litter size results from the greater total placental mass of animals carrying large litters. However, it remains to be determined whether the effect of litter size is due solely to an increase in the total number of mPL-II producing cells or whether the rate at which individual cells secrete mPL-II is also affected. The genotype of the feto-placental unit is important in determining both the gestational serum profile and the absolute concentration of mPL-II in the maternal serum. When female mice of the C3H\HeN strain were bred to BALB\c males, the gestational maternal serum mPL-II profile was similar to that of BALB\c females mated with BALB\c males, and the absolute concentration of mPL-II is serum was higher in females bred to males of a different strain than in females bred to males of the same strain (32). The pituitary exerts an inhibitory control over the maternal serum mPL-II concentration. Hypophysectomy of mice on day 10 of pregnancy or later resulted in a large increase in maternal serum mPL-II within 24 hours, and this increase was sustained for the remainder of pregnancy (7). The post-hypophysectomy rise in maternal serum of mPL-II could be suppressed by administration of mGH but not mPRL (17). Whether mGH regulates mPL-II such concentrations by acting directly at the placenta or indirectly via other organs such as the ovaries is still unknown. Treatment of mouse placental explants with progesterone *in vitro* inhibited the secretion of mPL-II (33). The development of an *in vitro* placental cell culture system (42) has allowed us to begin characterizing an mPL-II secretagogue which is produced by the decidua. An early hypothesis for the function of PLs, particularly human placental lactogen, proposed that the hormones may have a role in regulating maternal intermediary metabolism in such a way as to insure the availability of nutrients for the fetus (13). This hypothesis predicts that PL concentration should increase when nutrient availability is low. In mice, fasting for 24-48 hours during the second half of pregnancy was accompanied by an increase int the maternal serum mPL-II concentration (11). The factors involved in regulating mPL-I have not yet been determined.

Biological Activity

Due to the structural similarities between PLs and PRL and GH, much of the studies carried out on the biological activity of the PLs has examined the PRL and GH-like effects of these hormones in a variety of both homologous and heterologous biological test systems. The biological activity of PLs have been examined relative to role in steroidogenesis, growth and regulation of intermediary metabolism and growth and differentiation of mammary tissue. During pregnancy growth and differentiation of the mammary gland is controlled by a complex interaction of a number of hormones and growth factors (41). One of the hormones that is essential for both normal growth and differentiation of the mammary gland is PRL or a PRL-like hormone (20,22). In the mouse, pituitary PRL circulates in high concentration in the first half of pregnancy but thereafter declines and remains at low level until just before parturition when a peak occurs in the serum (38). In the latter half of pregnancy, PL-I and PL-II are the predominant PRL-DiKe lactogens in the circulation (24,30). Similar profiles for these placental lactogens are observed in both the hamster (37) and rat (26). Based on the structural similarities between the pituitary and placental hormones and their unique circulating profiles, we speculated that the PLs are the important lactogenic hormones in the latter half of pregnancy. While receptor studies for PRL, PL-I and PL-II in the mouse mammary gland have not yet been done, receptor studies utilizing ovarian and hepatic tissue would strongly suggest that these hormones all act through binding to the same receptors (15,21). *In vitro* studies have shown that both mPL-I and mPL-II are potent stimulators of alpha-lactalbumin production from cultured mouse mammary epithelial cells (6,40). Hamster PL-II has also been shown to lactogenic in mouse mammary tissue (34). Further evidence for the importance of PLs in the development of the mammary gland in rodents have come from *in vivo* studies. Early studies in both mice and rats showed that hypophysectomy during pregnancy in these species did not prevent mammary development when assessed at parturition (27,28). Subsequent studies (1) showed that mammary gland growth (estimated by DNA content) is not reduced just prior to parturition in rats that were hypophysectomized at days 11 to 15 of gestation provided that these animals carried 3 or more conceptuses. Likewise, we have recently found that mammary gland growth is comparable in intact mice and mice hypophysectomized at midgestation when assessed at day 14 and 18 of gestation (43). There was, however, significant reduction in the total RNA and alpha-lactalbumin content of the mammary gland of these hypophysectomized mice. Not surprisingly, hypophysectomy also caused a significant reduction of other circulating hormones that are important for the differentiation of the mammary gland. We feel that the lack of differentiation of the mammary gland in the hypophysectomized mice is not caused by the absence of PRL-like hormones from the pituitary, since PLs, potent lactogenic hormones, are found in high concentrations during the latter half of gestation. The reduction in the differentiation of the mammary gland in hypophysectomized mice was due to the lack of an interaction of all the hormones needed for this complex process. In studies recently initiated in our laboratory we are replacing the hormones that are affected by hypophysectomy. Preliminary studies have shown that administration of corticosterone and thyroxine simultaneously fully restores alpha-lactalbumin content in hypophysectomized mice. It is hoped that these studies will eventually allow us to determine how mouse PLs directly contribute to mammary gland growth and differentiation.

PLs in rodents have also been implicated as important luteotropins in the latter half of pregnancy. So far, a direct evidence for the role of mouse PLs in the maintenance of the corpus luteum is lacking. Our recent study (21) on the binding of mPL-I and mPL-II to mouse ovarian plasma membranes from different days of pregnancy provide evidence that these hormones are probably very important in stimulating ovarian processes during the latter half of pregnancy in the mouse.

PLs have also been implicated as having roles in growth and metabolism. In the mouse, while fasting has been shown to elevate mPL-II and circulating free fatty acids (11), we were unable to demonstrate any direct effect of mPL-II on lipolysis (12). Studies are underway to characterize in depth the biological function of mPL-I and mPL-II on tissues such as the liver, ovary and mammary gland.

Acknowledgments

We are extremely grateful to the many talented undergraduates, graduate students and postdoctoral fellows who have made major contributions to our research on placental lactogens. I (F.T.) wish to thank my Ph.D. supervisor, Professor Howard Bern for his continuous moral support; he indeed has been a major role model. The research described in this manuscript was supported by NSF grant PCM-8217382 and NIH grants HD 14966 and RR 08132.

References

1. Anderson, R. R., Mammary gland growth in the hypophysectomized pregnant rat, Proc. Soc. Exp. Biol. Med., 148:283 (1975).
2. Campbell, W. J., Deb, S., Kwok, S. C. M., Joslin, J. A., and Soares, M. J., Differential expression of placental lactogen-II and prolactin-like protein-A in the rat chorioallantoic placenta, Endocrinology, 125:1565 (1989).
3. Colosi, P., Marr, G., Lopez, J., Haro, L., Ogren, L., and Talamantes, F., Isolation, purification and characterization of mouse placental lactogen, Proc. Nat. Acad. Sci., 79:771 (1982).
4. Colosi, P., Ogren, L., Thordarson, G., and Talamantes, F., Purification and partial characterization of two prolactin-like glycoprotein hormones from the midpregnant mouse conceptus, Endocrinology, 120:2500 (1987).
5. Colosi, P., Talamantes, F., and Linzer, D. I. H., Molecular cloning, characterization and expression of mPL-I cDNA, Mol. Endocrinol., 1:767 (1987).
6. Colosi, P., Ogren, L., Southard, J., Thordarson, G., Linzer, D. I. H., and Talamantes, F., Biological, immunological and binding properties of recombinant mouse placental lactogen-I, Endocrinology, 123:2662 (1988).
7. Day, J., Ogren, L., and Talamantes, F., The effect of hypophysectomy on serum placental lactogen and progesterone in the mouse, Endocrinology, 119:898 (1986).
8. Duckworth, M. L., Kirk, K. L., and Friesen, H. G. l, Isolation and identification of a cDNA clone of rat placental lactogen II, J. Biol. Chem., 261:10871 (1986).
9. Duckworth, M. L., Peden, L. M., and Friesen, H. G., Isolation of a novel prolactin-like cDNA clone from developing rat placenta, J. Biol. Chem., 261:10879 (1986).
10. Duckworth, M. L., Peden, L. M., and Friesen, H. G., A third prolactin-like protein expressed by the developing rat placenta: complementary deoxyribonucleic aced sequence and partial structure of the gene, Mol. Endocrinol., 2:912 (1988).
11. Fielder, P. J., Ogren, L., Edwards, D., and Talamantes, F., Effects of fasting on serum lactogenic hormone concentrations during mid and late pregnancy in mice, Am. J. Physiol. (Endocrinol. Metab.) 16:40 (1987).
12. Fielder, P. J. and Talamantes, F., The lipolytic effects of mPL-II, mPRL and mGH on virgin and pregnant mouse adipose tissue. Endocrinology, 121:493 (1987).
13. Grumbach, M. M., Kaplan, S. L., Sciarra, J. J., and Burr, I. M., Chorionic growth hormone-prolactin (CGP): secretion, disposition, biological activity in man and postulated function as the "growth hormone" of the second half of pregnancy. Ann NY Acad. Sci., 148:501 (1986).
14. Hall, J. and Talamantes, F., Immunocytochemical localization of mouse placental lactogen in the mouse placenta, J. Histochem. Cytochem., 32:379 (1984).
15. Harigaya, T., Smith, W. C., and Talamantes, F., Hepatic placental lactogen receptors during pregnancy in the mouse. Endocrinology, 122:1366 (1988).
16. Jackson, L. L., Colosi, P., Talamantes, F., and Linzer, D. I. H., Molecular cloning of mouse placental lactogen cDNA, Proc. Natl. Acad. Sci. 83:8496 (1986).
17. Kishi, K., Ogren, L., Southard, J. N., and Talamantes, F., Pituitary factors regulating mouse placental lactogen-II (mPL-II) secretion during the last half of pregnancy in mice. Endocrinology 122:2309 (1988).
18. Linzer, D. I. H., Lee, S. E., Ogren, L., Talamantes, F., and Nathans, D., Identification of proliferin RNA and protein in mouse placenta. Proc. Natl. Acad. Sci. 82:4356 (1985).
19. Linzer, D. I. H. and Nathans, D., A new member of the prolactin-growth hormone gene family expressed in mouse placenta, EMBO J., 4:1419 (1985).
20. Lyons, W. R., Li, C. H., and Johnson, R. E., The hormonal control of mammary growth and lactation, Recent Prog. Horm. Res. 14:219 (1958).
21. MacLeod, K. R., Smith, W. C., Ogren, L., and Talamantes, F., Recombinant mouse placental lactogen-I binds to lactogen receptors in mouse liver and ovary: partial characterization of the ovarian receptor. Endocrinology, 125:2258 (1989).
22. Nandi, S., Endocrine control of mammary-gland development and function in the C3H\He Crgl mouse, J. Natl. Cancer Inst.,21:1039 (1958).

23. Ogren, L. and Talamantes, F., Prolactins of pregnancy and their cellular source. In: *The International Review of Cytology, Vol. 12*, H. Bourne, (ed.), New York, Academic Press, (1988).

24. Ogren, L., Southard, J. N., Colosi, P., Linzer, D. I. H., and Talamantes, F., Mouse placental lactogen-I:RIA and gestational profile in maternal serum, Endocrinology, 125:2253 (1989).

25. Pinon, I., Kishi, K., and Talamantes, F., The kinetics of disappearance of endogenous mouse placental lactogen-II in intact and hypophysectomized pregnant mice, Mol. Cell. Endocrinol., 55:45 (1988).

26. Robertson, M. D. and Friesen, H. G., Two forms of rat placental lactogen revealed by radioimmunoassay, Endocrinology, 108:2388 (1981).

27. Selye, H., Collip, J. B., and Thompson, D. L., Effect of hypophysectomy upon pregnancy and lactation, Proc. Soc. Exp. Biol. Med., 31:82 (1934).

28. Selye, H., Collip, J. B., and Thompson, D. L., Effect of hypophysectomy upon pregnancy and lactation, Proc. Soc. Exp. Biol. Med., 30:589 (1933).

29. Schuler, L. and Hurley, W. L., Molecular cloning of a prolactin-related mRNA expressed in bovine placenta. Proc. Natl. Acad. Sci. 84:5650 (1987).

30. Soares, M. J. and Talamantes, F., The development and characterization of a homologous radioimmunoassay for mouse placental lactogen, Endocrinology, 110:668 (1982).

31. Soares, M. J., Colosi, P, Thordarson, G., and Talamantes, F., Identification and partial characterization of a lactogen from the midpregnant mouse conceptus, Endocrinology, 12:1313 (1983).

32. Soares, M. J. and Talamantes, F., Genetic and litter size effects on serum placental lactogen in the mouse, Biol. Reprod., 29:165 (1983).

33. Soares, M. J. and Talamantes, F., Placental lactogen secretion in the mouse: *In vitro* responses and ovarian hormonal influences, J. Exper. Zool., 234:97 (1985).

34. Southard, J. N., Thordarson, G., and Talamantes, F., Purification and characterization of hamster placental lactogen. Endocrinology 119:508 (1986).

35. Southard, J. and Talamantes, F., Immunological studies of rodent placental lactogens, Mol. Cell. Endocrinol., 50:29 (1987).

36. Southard, J. N., Do, L., Smith, W. C., and Talamantes, F., Hamster placental lactogen-II contains a structural feature unique among the growth hormone-prolactin-placental lactogen family, Mol. Endocrinol., 3:1710 (1989).

37. Southard, J. N., Campbell, G. T., and Talamantes, F., Hamster placental lactogens: gestational profiles and high molecular weight forms. Endocrinology 121:900 (1987).

38. Talamantes, F., Soares, M. J., Colosi, P., Haro, L., and Ogren, L., The biochemistry and physiology of mouse placental lactogen. In: *Prolactin Secretion: A Multidisciplinary Approach*, F. Mena and C. M. Valverde-R, (eds.), New York, Academic Press, (1984).

39. Talamantes, F. and Ogren, L., The placenta as an endocrine organ: polypeptides. In: *The Physiology of Reproduction*, E. Knobil and J. Neil, (eds.), New York, Raven Press, LTD, (1987).

40. Thordarson, G., Villalobos, R., Colosi, P., Southard, J., Ogren, L., and Talamantes, F., The lactogenic response of cultured mouse mammary epithelial cells to mouse placental lactogen, J. Endocrinol., 109:263 (1986).

41. Thordarson, G. and Talamantes, F., *Role of the Placenta in Mammary Gland Development and Function*, M. C. Neville and C. Daniel, (eds.), New York, Plenum Press, (1987).

42. Thordarson, G., Folger, P., and Talamantes, F., Development of a placental cell culture system for studying the control of mouse placental lactogen secretion, Placenta, 8:573 (1987).

43. Thordarson, G., Ogren, L., Day, J. R., Bowens, K., Fielder, P., and Talamantes, F., Mammary gland development and alpha-lactalbumin production in hypophysectomized, pregnant mice, Biol. Reprod., 40:517 (1989).

Questions

Dr. Bern: If I could go back to the very beginning of your talk on the structure of placental lactogens. The prolactin molecule and the placental lactogen molecule. It appears that there may be different effects of teleost prolactin and that of the tetrapods. Could any of these differences be due to structural or secondary differences in these molecules?

Dr. Talamantes: I think that studies such as to those by Dan Linser using site-specific mutagenesis is really going to be able to answer that question because he is able to take mouse placental lactogen (mpl) and mouse prolactin, and he's able to perform site specific mutagenesis. There was a theory by Baxter and others on the evolution of placental lactogens. This was based on the structure of human placental lactogen. Hpl has approximately 96% sequence homology with human growth hormone and it doesn't have a lot of growth promoting activity and the evolution turns out to be very different than the evolution of the other placental lactogens. It's interesting that the hamster placental lactogen has the three disulfide loops. But now we know that when you take mouse placental lactogen II or rat placental lactogen II and add it to serum and chromatograph it, we would never see these large forms of the molecule like we saw in the hamster. Some thought it was a nonspecific effect. It turns out that the presence of this extra loop at the amino terminus of the hamster placenta lactogen may well account for the sulfide bonding to the serum protein. It now appears that these polypeptide hormones such as growth hormone and placental lactogen have binding proteins just like the steroid hormones. Thus it may be that these loops have different functions which people simply haven't thought about. What we plan to do now is to use cDNAs to put an extra loop in the mpl II and see if that will help them bind to the complexes.

Dr. Bern: How many loops does ovine PLII have?

Dr. Talamantes: I think it has three loops.

12

The Origin and Role of Cytokines Determining Success and Failure in the Post-Implantation Period

David A. Clark
McMaster University
Department of Medicine
Hamilton, Ontario, Canada

Introduction

The success of mammalian pregnancy is believed to depend on a co-ordinated sequence of synchronized events in the uterus and in the embryo. For example, loss of appropriate phasing between developmental events in the pre-implantation embryo and uterus may account for implantation failure of *in vitro* fertilized oocytes in the rat (1) and with *in vivo* embryo transfer in domestic animals (2). One may view the normal co-ordination of events simply as a manifestation of the independent execution of a genetically defined program which achieves its synchrony when the "seed" and the "soil" belong to the same species. However, there is increasing evidence of an interplay between the embryo and the uterus whereby signals pass from one to the other. The success of pregnancy may then depend upon successful co-operation.

Co-ordination in multicellular organisms depends on inter-cellular communication. The most primitive mechanism is that of cell-cell contact whereby interaction between a ligand on the surface of one cell with a receptor on a second cell alters the behavior of one or both of the parties. Formation of gap junctions between cells may also permit the passage of informational signals from cell to cell (3). A second level of communication may be achieved via metabolic gradients or gradients of small molecules such as the prostaglandin-leukotriene-eicosinoids and other autocoids such as histamine and serotonin (4-9). Long distance communication becomes essential in large multicellular bodies is achieved by specialized cells with long processes which extend over long distances (i.e. nerves) and signal their target by local release of neurotransmitters. Alternately, long-distance messages may be sent via the circulatory system as exemplified by the endocrine system. Here, the message is a soluble hormone which is produced by a specialized cell type (usually localized in a endocrine gland) and binds to specific receptors in the cells of the target tissue altering its function. Intermediate between localized neurotransmitters and circulating hormones there are cytokines, small polypeptides that may be produced by a variety of cells and which exert pleiotropic effects, either stimulating or inhibiting the target cell (10).

Figure 1 illustrates the time of occurrence of a variety of cytokines during several stages of early pregnancy when failure in the form of infertility, occult pregnancy loss, and clinical miscarriage may occur. Polypeptide cytokines are shown in bold face and other non-polypeptide small molecular mediators in italics. Cytokines such as interleukin 1 and tumor necrosis factor-alpha (TNF-a) produced by macrophages in peritoneal fluid of patients with endometriosis (and possibly also unexplained infertility (31,32,33)) and thought to cause implantation failure are not included as these cytokines are not part of the pathophysiology of abnormal rather than normal pregnancy. The remainder of this chapter will deal with the problem of failure after implantation and the possible role that cytokines may play in

Cellular Signals Controlling Uterine Function
Edited by L.A. Lavia, Plenum Press, New York

determining success or failure. In this respect, I have designated a peri-implantation phase of early trophoblast invasion and induction of decidualization as separate from a post-implantation phase where a distinct fetus and placenta form. From the standpoint of investigating the problem of human pregnancy failure we are dependent upon clues from the study of animal systems and in this regard most of the data has been obtained from studying spontaneous abortion in mice. This event usually occurs in the post-implantation period illustrated in Figure 1 and is most often seen as a resorption without external expulsion of products of conception. The similarity of resorption to clinically evident spontaneous abortion in humans is argued elsewhere (34).

Several murine models of spontaneous abortion have been described (34,35) but the most extensively investigated is the system in which inbred females of the CBA/J strain are bred to DBA/2 or DBA/1 males. Here the male and female differ at a number of genetic loci including the major histocompatibility complex (H-2 in the mouse). Pregnancy failure is therefore not a manifestation of further inbreeding (indeed, one would expect "hybrid vigor" to result in a large litter) and the occurrence of spontaneous abortion in an outbred mating situation is similar to reproduction in the human population. A second feature of the CBA-DBA/2 system is the resorption rate increases with age (36) and this is also seen in the human. In the aged CBA mouse, post-implantation loss is not corrected by administration of gestational hormones (37). A third feature is that the resorptions are recurrent and can be prevented by immunizing the CBA/J females against the H-2^d antigens of the DBA/2 male before mating (36,38) and there is parallel evidence to suggest immunization may partially prevent human recurrent abortion (39). Investigation of the mechanisms underlying pregnancy failure in the CBA-DBA system and its treatment by immunotherapy is therefore highly relevant to problems in humans.

Initially it was suspected that spontaneous abortion in allopregnant CBA/J mice might be due to rejection of the "fetal allograft." The reasoning was as follows. First, both the fetus and its trophoblast express antigens against which the maternal immune system can (and often does) react. Some of these antigens are strong transplantation antigens inherited from the father such as Class I MHC (major histocompatibility complex) antigens (40) recognizable by maternal cytotoxic T lymphocytes (CTL). Second, class I paternal MHC is expressed on the mouse placenta at about the time of onset of spontaneous abortion (41). Third, there is a maternal cellular infiltrate into the placenta and aborting fetus and maternal cytotoxic T cells against Class 1 paternal MHC can be isolated from resorption tissue. (36,38).Fourth, during normal successful pregnancy, a novel type of non-thymus dependent lymphocytic suppressor cell accumulates in maternal decidua at the implantation site in response to soluble signals from the fetal trophoblast (37,42,43). These suppressor cells release a potent suppressor factor related to transforming growth factor-beta (beta 2 type) that blocks the response of CTL to the cytokine interleukin 2 (IL-2) that is produced by T cells at the site of allograft rejection (17,44,45). Indeed, IL-2 is a key cytokine in allograft rejection and blocking IL-2 production or action also inhibits graft rejection (45,46). Interestingly, the suppressor cell activity in decidua developed at the same time as expression of Class 1 antigens on placenta and a deficiency of suppressor activity predicted which embryos would subsequently abort (36). Fifth, immunization against abortion (which is mediated by an MHC-antigen-specific molecule in serum, presumably antibody) boosted the level of suppressor cell activity without significantly affecting systemic CTL responses (47,48). Taken together, these data supported a model wherein abortion was prevented by local active suppression of maternal CTL activity and where antibody responses acted to enhance graft survival by boosting suppressor cell activity.

Recent experimental data have exposed some flaws in the above synthesis and have led to a major revision of the rejection model of abortion. First, class 1 MHC-bearing trophoblast cells are highly resistant to lysis by CTL (49). Second,*in vivo* injection of antibody to deplete T cells or to block the IL-2 receptor does not decrease the rate of abortion significantly (38,50,51). Third, *in vivo* injection of antibody against the asialo-GM1

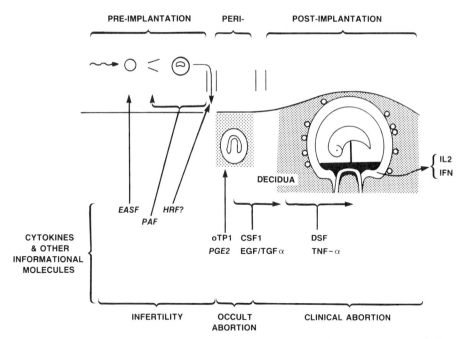

Figure 1. Time of appearance and action of cytokines and other small informational molecules during early pregnancy. Non-cytokine molecules in italics include EASF (embryo-associated suppressor factor)(11), PAF (platelet activating factor), HRF (histamine releasing factor)(9), PGE2 (prostaglandin E2)(4,7). Cytokine polypeptides include the embryo-derived interferon α2-like oTP1 that acts on decidua to inhibit production of PGF2a (13), uterine epithelial CSF1 (14), EGF/TGF-α (epidermal growth factor/transforming growth factor-alpha)(15,16), DSF (decidual suppressor factor)(17) and TNF-α(tumor necrosis factor-alpha)(18,19). Other decidua-derived such as IGF1 (insulin-like growth factor-1)(20), prolactin (21), and IL-1 (22) are not illustrated due to lack of data on their kinetics. The placenta may produce IL-2 (interleukin 2)(23) and interferon (13,24) as illustrated. Other placental cytokines not shown include IL-1 (25), GM-CSF (26), placental lactogens and proliferin/prolactins (29,30).

determinant reduces the abortion rate (52,53). Asialo-GM1 is a cell surface marker found on about 1/2 of natural killer cells and on lymphokine activated killer cells (LAKs). Trophoblast cells appear sensitive to lysis by LAKs (54).

LAKs and NK cells belong to the para-immunological innate resistance system (illustrated in Figure 2) that is spontaneously active and selectively kills primitive embryonic-type cells such as tumor cells and virally-altered and transformed cells. The natural effector system is thus able to reject grafts of small numbers of cells rapidly and without the delay inherent in antigen-specific immune responses. The natural effector system also includes macrophages and natural cytotoxic cells (NC)(not shown). Macrophages are present in the murine uterus during pregnancy and can release cytokines such as tumor necrosis factor-alpha (TNF-a)(53). TNF-α can cause death of non-antigenic tumor grafts by thrombosing the vascular supply (55). TNF-α can also participate in the activation of LAKs (as illustrated in Figure 2)(56,57) and can bind to receptors on trophoblast (58) (effect unknown). It should also be recalled from Figure 1 that placental cells (including trophoblast) appears to produce cytokines such as IL-2 and interferon (an activator of NK cells)(13,22,24); IL-2 and TNF-α may be synergistic in LAK activation in some systems (57). Taken together these data have led to the hypothesis that there is deliberate activation of natural effector cells in decidua by the conceptus the purpose of which may be to eliminate embryos not sufficiently healthy to be able to activate non-T suppressor cells at the implantation site (54). Some recent data relevant to testing this hypothesis will now be presented.

Materials and Methods

Mice used, procedure for mating and uterine cell harvest, preparation of supernatants from decidua, and tissue culture assay for suppression of CTL generation have been described in detail elsewhere (17,36). The Be6 murine placental cell line with trophoblastic features and its use in an assay for killing by LAK effector cells (or by TNF-a) was done as described (59) and inhibition of proliferation was tested by tritiated thymidine uptake after 48 hrs of culture (5 x 10^3 cells plated/well). *In vivo* treatments with rabbit anti-asialo GM1 (or normal rabbit serum control) was done on day 6.5-7.5 or days 9.5-10.5 of pregnancy (52). Assay for TNF-α activity was done using a 1/4 dilution of decidual supernatant incubated with ^{51}Cr-labelled WEHI-164 target cells for 20 hrs at 37·C and a standard curve generated using recombinant TNF-a.

Generation of anti-Be6 LAK effectors was performed in a microculture system (44,53) substituting cytokines for F1 stimulatory cells. Decidual suppressor factor was HPLC purified as described elsewhere (17).

Results and Discussion

Release of cytokines from the decidua of DBA/2-mated CBA/J mice with a high rate of abortion beginning day 10.5 was compared to the pattern of low abortion C3H/HeJ mice. By day 10.5, release of soluble TGF-β2-related suppressor factor occurred from C3H decidua whereas release was delayed and lower in activity when decidua from the aborting mice was used. Conversely, the aborting mice showed an accelerated appearance of the ability to release TNF-α that paralleled the onset of abortion. TNF-α levels were also higher in CBA than in C3H. It has been shown that administration of TNF-α to allopregnant CBA/J mice increases the abortion rate (53,60) and conversely, pentoxyphylene, an inhibitor of TNF-a, decreases the abortion rate (M. Baines, personal communication, manuscript submitted for publication). Injection of LPS into low abortion type females such as C3H stimulates TNF-α release and abortion (60,61). It therefore appears that TNF-α may be a critical mediator of the abortion process in CBA/J mice.

To further investigate possible mechanisms of TNF-a-mediated abortion, some comparisons were made between the decidua associated with aborting vs non-aborting sites.

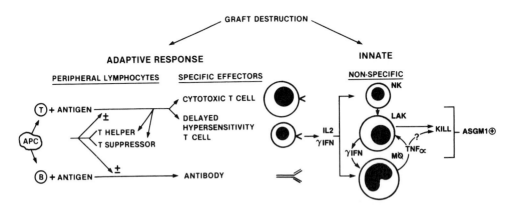

Figure 2. Simple illustration of the cellular systems responsible for host resistance to various types of grafts. The specific immune system is responsible for antigen-specific adaptive responses whereas the innate system or natural resistance system acts selectively against certain types of primitive cells. Components of the innate system relevant to the discussion in this paper are shown.

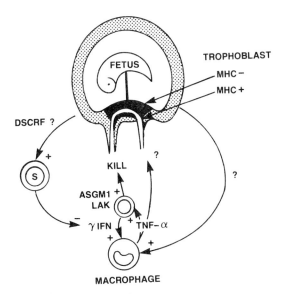

Figure 3. A model of the cellular interactions determining the balance between survival or abortion during the post-implantation phase of pregnancy in the mouse. DSCRF (decidual suppressor cell recruiting factor) represents a demonstrated activity (43) the molecular nature of which is still unknown. For possible candidates see legend to Figure 1.

Injection of asialo-GM1 antibody reduced the abortion rate even when given as late as day 10.5 but the treatment did <u>not</u> reduce production of TNF-a. Further, when supernatants from aborting and non-aborting sites were compared, no difference in TNF-α activity was detected. The ability of TNF-α to damage the Be6 trophoblast cell line was tested. Only very high levels of recombinant TNF-α produced lysis (10 units/ml or more), lower concentrations inhibited proliferation, but the levels of TNF-α obtained from decidua at the time of abortion in CBA/J mice were below the minimum inhibitory level. It therefore seemed unlikely that TNF-α was acting as a direct cytotoxin. Indeed, the main difference between resorption and healthy implant sites was lower suppressor activity associated with supernatants from resorption sites and the presence of effector cells in the implant site decidua capable of killing Be6 target cells *in vitro* at effector-to-target ratios of 3:1-12:1. Interestingly, this killer cell activity could be depleted by treatment with anti-asialo GM1. These data suggested that either the TGF-β2-related decidual suppressor cytokine was protecting the pregnancy from some unidentified effects of TNF-α on trophoblast or the vasculature, or that the suppressor cytokine was inhibiting the activation of anti-trophoblast killer cells (by TNF-α ± IL-2) at healthy implant sites.

Several additional experimental observations suggest the latter may be correct. First, anti-Be6 killer cells could be generated *in vitro* in response to IL2 and/or TNF-a, even when spleen cells from SCID mice lacking T and B lymphocytes were used (53). Second, spontaneous abortion was enhanced following daily *in vivo* injection of the 7D4 monoclonal anti-IL-2 receptor antibody. This antibody does not block allograft rejection or binding of IL-2 to its receptor, but under dilute conditions, enhances the generation of anti-Be6 killer cells (35,53). Third, purified decidual suppressor factor inhibited the generation of anti-Be6 LAKs but had little effect on TNF-α production *in vitro* (53 and manuscript in preparation). Fourth, it has been reported that only a proportion of implantation sites in DBA/2-mated CBA/J mice show an infiltration with asialo-GM1+ cells (62) and it is therefore proposed that these are sites with suppressor factor deficiency that allow the asialo-GM1+ precursors of LAKs to become activated when TNF-α levels rise.

There are some important issues raised by observation (d). The cellular infiltrate of asialo-GM1+ cells occurs by day 6.5 of pregnancy and what determines whether or not an implant site will be infiltrated is unclear. Since suppressor cell activity in decidua at the time of onset of abortion (after day 9.5) is dependent upon trophoblast, one could suspect that the asialo-GM1+ cells might themselves compromise trophoblast development and thereby produce implant sites deficient in suppressor activity. If cellular infiltration at day 9.5 and low suppression were independently determined, the proportion of sites that abort would have to be much lower than the proportion of sites (30 %) with infiltrates and this is contrary to current data (51,62). If the asialo-GM1+ cell present in decidua prior to abortion caused low levels of suppression at involved sites, treatment with asialo-GM1 should increase soluble suppressor activity per uterus. Some increase in activity was noted, compatible with an increased proportion of non-resorbing sites per uterus.

Our current hypothesis concerning abortion in the CBA-DBA/2 system is as follows. First, inadequate development of trophoblast-dependent suppressor cell activity is related to a cellular infiltrate by asialo-GM1+ cells, susceptibility to which is determined by events in the peri-implantation phase of pregnancy. In this regard it is interesting that transfer of protection against abortion by anti-H-2^d (MHC) antibody only occurs if the antibody is given during or prior to the peri-implant phase and that immunization acts to block the infiltrate of asialo-GM1+ cells. Further, in peri-implant decidua there is a different type of suppressor cell to that found in the post-implant period. The latter is a small non-T lymphocytic cell dependent upon trophoblast whereas the peri-implant suppressor cell is a large hormone-dependent cell bearing the CD8 T cell marker does not release a detectable soluble suppressor factor!(51) *In vivo* depletion of this CD8+ cell during the peri-implant period leads to a marked increase in the abortion rate (51). Since antigen-antibody complexes are known to be able to activate CD8+ suppressor T cells (63), it is reasonable to hypothesize that anti-H2^d antibody acts in CD8+ cells that then block the infiltration by asialo-GM1+ cells. How might this CD8+ cell act? We have also found that a single low dose of GM-CSF given on day 7.5 of CBA-DBA/2 pregnancy can prevent abortion, and protection can be achieved using cytokines that lack trophoblast stimulating activity but which can inhibit the generation of anti-Be6 killer cells (53,64). Immunization against abortion increases GM-CSF levels in decidua (60,65). It is therefore suspected that CD8+ cells may release CSF-like factors that play a dual role in stimulating trophoblast (minor role) and in inhibiting the local accumulation of asialo-GM1+ cells (major role). A deficiency of CD8+ cell-dependent functions would lead to retarded trophoblast development and presence of asialo-GM1+ cells. Later during pregnancy, the asialo-GM1+ cells would become activated to cytotoxicity by TNF-α and kill any trophoblast undefended by TGF-β2 related DSF. In the absence of TNF-α and asialo-GM1+ cells, abortion does not occur. Figure 3 illustrates the proposal of interactions. Second, the accelerated rise in TNF-α production that occurs in CBA/J mice does not appear specific for a subset of implantation sites. It does appear specific for a particular phase of pregnancy and likely arises from macrophages in response to the conceptus. When TNF-α levels rise, implants with asialo-GM1+ infiltrates will be killed. Whether CBAxDBA/2 pregnancy is unique in showing an accelerated production of TNF-α is unclear. Abortion in the CBA/J mouse is dependent upon a normal flora (66), and this may play a role in activating macrophages to respond with greater TNF-α production when triggered in the uterus.

It is no doubt clear to the perceptive reader that many key details concerning cellular and cytokine-dependent events in the above processes remain to be verified by experimental data. Nevertheless, further efforts to dissect the underlying mechanisms are being pursued, and one's enthusiasm for the task is enhanced by parallel studies we have done using decidua from early human spontaneous abortions where a deficiency of suppressor cell and suppressor factor activity (67,68) as has been documented similar to the findings in the spontaneously aborting CBA/J mouse.

150

Acknowledgments

Supported by grants from MRC Canada (MA9707, MT6447) and by an MRC Scientist career award.

References

1. Venderhyden, B. C., Rouleau, A., Walton, E. A., and Armstrong, D. T., Increased mortality during early embryonic development after *in vitro* fertilization of rat oocytes, J. Reprod. Fert. 77:401 (1986).
2. Pope, W. F., Uterine asynchrony: a cause of embryonic loss, Biol. Reprod. 39:999 (1988).
3. Winterhager, E., Brümmer, F., Dermietzel, R., Hülser, D. F., and Denker, H.-W., Gap junction formation in rabbit uterine epithelium in response to embryo recognition, Develop. Biol. 126:203 (1988).
4. Tawfik, O. W., Sagrillo, C., Johnson, D. C., and Dey, S. K., Decidualization in the rat: role of leukotrienes and prostaglandins, Prostagland. Leuk. Medicine 29:221 (1987).
5. Gupta, A., Huet, Y. M., and Dey, S. K., Evidence for prostaglandins and leukotrienes as mediators of phase I of estrogen action in implantation in the mouse, Endocrinol. 124:546 (1989).
6. Aliverti, V., Bonanomi, L., Giavini, E., Leone, V. G., Mariani, L., Prati, M. and Vismara, C., Embryotoxic effects of 5-hydroxytryptamine during the peri-implantation period in the rat, Biol. Reprod. 27:1231 (1982).
7. Kennedy, T. G., Intrauterine infusion of prostaglandins and decidualization in rats with uteri differentially sensitized for the decidual cell reaction, Biol. Reprod. 34:327 (1986).
8. Mitchell, J. A. and Hammer, R. E., Serotonin-induced disruption of implantation in the rat: I. Serum progesterone, implantation site blood flow, and intrauterine $p0_2$, Biol. Reprod. 28:830 (1983).
9. Cocchiara, R., Di Trapani, G., Azzolina, A., Albeggiani, G., and Geraci, D., Identification of a histamine-releasing factor secreted by human pre-implantation embryos grown *in vitro*, J. Reprod. Immunol. 13:41 (1988).
10. Sporn, M. B. and Roberts, A. B., Peptide growth factors are multifunctional, Nature 332:217 (1988).
11. Clark, D. A., Lee, S., Fishell, S., Mahadevan, M., Goodall, H., Ah Moye, M., Schechter, O., Stedronska-Clark, J., Underwood, J., Craft, I. and Mowbray, J., Immunosuppressive activity in human *in vitro* fertilization (IVF) culture supernatants and prediction of the outcome of embryo transfer: a multicenter trial, J. *In vitro* Fert. Embryo Transfer 6:51 (1989).
12. Spinks, N. R. and O'Neill, C., Embryo-derived platelet-activating factor essential for establishment of pregnancy in the mouse, Lancet 1:106 (1987).
13. Roberts, R. M., A novel group of interferons associated with the early ovine and bovine embryo, J. Interferon Res. 9:373 (1989).
14. Pollard, J. W., Bartocci, A., Arceci, R., Orlofsky, A., Ladner, M. B. and Stanley, E. R., Apparent role of the macrophage growth factor, CSF-1, in placental developments, Nature 330:484 (1987).
15. Brown, M., Zogg, J. L., Schultz, G. S., and Hilton, F. K., Increased binding of epidermal growth factor at preimplantation sites in mouse uteri, Endocrinol. 124:2882 (1989).
16. Morrish, D. W., Bhardwaj, D., Dabbagh, L. K., Marusyk, H., and Siy, O., Epidermal growth factor induces differentiation and secretion of human chorionic gonadotrophin and placental lactogen in normal human placenta, J. Clin. Endocrinol. Metab. 65:1282 (1987).
17. Clark, D. A., Falbo, M., Rowley, R. B., Banwatt, D., and Stedronska-Clark, J., Active suppression of host-versus-graft reaction in pregnant mice. IX. Soluble suppressor activity obtained from allopregnant mouse decidua that blocks the response to interleukin 2 is related to TGF-β, J. Immunol. 141:3833 (1988).

18. Jäättelä, M., Kuusela, P., and Saksela, E., Demonstration of tumor necrosis factor in human amniotic fluids and supernatants of placental and decidual tissues, Lab. Invest. 58:48 (1988).

19. Clark, D. A., Banwatt, D., Manuel, J., and Fulop, G., Cytokines and natural effector cells in successful and abortive pregnancies in immunodeficient SCID and DBA2-mated CBA/J mice, J. Reprod. Immunol. Suppl.1:83 (1989).

20. Murphy, L. J., Murphy, L. C., and Friesen, H. G., Estrogen induces insulin-like growth factor-I expression in the rat uterus, Molec. Endocrinol. 1:445 (1987).

21. Thrailkill, K. M., Golander, A., Underwood, L. E., and Handwerger, S., Insulin-like growth factor I stimulates the synthesis and release of prolactin from human decidual cells, Endocrinol. 123:2930 (1988).

22. Romero, R., Wu, Y. K., Brody, D. T., Oyarzum, E., Duff, G. W., and Durum, S. K., Human decidua: a source of interleukin-1, Obstet. Gynecol. 73:31 (1989).

23. Boehm, K., Kelley, M. F., Ilan, J., and Ilan, J., The interleukin 2 gene is expressed in the syncytiotrophoblast of the human placenta, Proc. Natl. Acad. Sci USA 866:656 (1989).

24. Fowler, A. K., Reed, C. D., and Giron, D. J., Identification of an interferon in murine placentas, Nature 286:266 (1980).

25. Flynn, A., Finke, J. H., and Loftus, M. A., Comparison of interleukin 1 production by adherent cells and tissue pieces from human placenta, Immunopharmacol. 9:19 (1985).

26. Cukrova, V. and Hrkal, Z., Purification and characterization of granulocyte-macrophage colony stimulating factor form human placenta. J. Chromatogr. 413:242 (1987).

27. Thordarson, G., Folger, P., and Talamantes, F., Development of a placental cell culture system for studying the control of mouse placental lactogen II secretion, Placenta 8:573 (1987).

28. Duckworth, M. L., Peden, L. M., and Friesen, H. G., A third prolactin-like protein expressed by the developing rat placenta: complementary deoxyribonucleic acid sequence and partial structure of the gene, Molec. Endocrinol. 2:912 (1988).

29. Miller, D. A., Lee, A., Pelton, R. W., Chen, E. Y., Moses, H. L., and Derynck, R., Murine transforming growth factor-$\beta 2$ cDNA sequence and expression in adult tissues and embryos, Molec. Endocrinol. 3:1108 (1989).

30. McLachlan, R. I., Healy, D. L., Robertson, D. M., Burger, H. G., and de Kretser, D.M., The human placenta: a novel source of inhibin, Biochem. Biophys. Res. Comm. 140:485 (1986).

31. Fakih, H., Baggett, B., Holtz, G., Tsang, K.-Y., Lee, J. C., and Williamson, H. O., Interleukin-1: a possible role in the infertility associated with endometriosis, Fertil. Steril. 47:213 (1987).

32. Eisermann, J., Gast, M. J., Pineda, J., Odem, R. R., and Collins, J. L., Tumor necrosis factor in peritoneal fluid of women undergoing laparoscopic surgery, Fertil. Steril. 50:573 (1988).

33. Hill, J. A., Faris, H. M., Schiff, I., and Anderson, D. J., Characterization of leukocyte subpopulations in the peritoneal fluid of women with endometriosis, Fertil. Steril. 50:216 (1988).

34. Clark, D. A., Animals models of early pregnancy loss. In: Immunologic Obstetrics, C. B. Coulamn, W. P. Faulk, and J. A. McIntyre (eds.), (in press).

35. Clark, D. A. and G. Chaouat. What do we know about spontaneous abortion mechanisms, Amer. J. Reprod. Immunol. Microbiol. 19:28 (1989).

36. Clark, D. A., Chaput, A., and Tutton, D., Active suppression of host-versus-graft reaction in pregnant mice. VII. Spontaneous abortion of allogeneic DBA/2 x CBA/J fetuses in the uterus of CBA/J mice correlates with deficient non-T suppressor cell activity, J. Immunol. 136:1668 (1986).

37. Gosden, R. G., Ovarian support of pregnancy in aging inbred mice, J. Reprod. Fert. 42:423 (1975).

38. Chaouat, G., Clark, D. A., and Wegmann, T. G., Genetic aspects of the CBA x DBA/2 and B10 x B10.A models of murine pregnancy failure and its prevention by lymphocyte

immunization. In: *Early Pregnancy Loss: Mechanisms and Treatment*, R. W. Beard and F. Sharp, (eds.), Ashton-under-Lyne, U.K., Peacock Press, p. 89 (1988).

39. Mowbray, J. F., Gibbings, C., Lindell, H., Reginald, P. W., Underwood, J. L., and Beard, R. W., Controlled trial of treatment of recurrent spontaneous abortion by immunization with paternal cells, Lancet 1:941 (1985).

40. Clark, D. A., Slapsys, R., Chaput, A., Walker, C., Brierley, J., Daya, S., and Rosenthan, K., Immunoregulatory molecules of trophoblast and decidual suppressor cell origin at the materno-fetal interface, Amer. J. Reprod. Immunol. Microbiol. 10:100 (1986).

41. Raghupathy, R., Singh, B., Barrington-Leigh, J., and Wegmann, T. G., Ontogeny and turnover kinetics of paternal H-2K antigenic determinants on the allogeneic murine placenta, J. Immunol. 127:2074 (1981).

42. Slapsys, R. M., Richards, C. D., and Clark, D. A., Active suppression of host-versus-graft reaction in pregnant mice. VIII. The uterine decidua-associated suppressor cell is distinct from decidual NK cells, Cell Immunol. 99:140 (1985).

43. Slapsys, R. M., Younglai, E., and Clark, D. A., A novel suppressor cell is recruited to decidua by fetal trophoblast-type cells, Reg. Immunol. 1:182 (1988).

44. Clark, D.A., Harley, C., Book, W., and Flanders, K., Suppressor factor in murine pregnancy decidua is related to transforming growth factor beta-2, FASEB J. 3:A503 (1989).

45. Espevik, T., Figari, I. A., Shalaby, M. R., Lackides, G. A., Lewis, G. D., Shepard, H. M., and Palladino, M. A., Jr., Inhibition of cytokine production by cyclosporin A and transforming growth factor β, J. Exp. Med. 166:571 (1987).

46. Kirkman, R. L., Barrett, L. V., Gaulton, G. N., Kelley, V. E., Ythier, A., and Strom, T. B., Administration of an anti-interleukin 2 receptor monoclonal antibody prolongs cardiac allograft survival in mice, J. Exp. Med. 162:358 (1985).

47. Clark, D. A., Kiger, N., Guenet, J. L., and Chaouat, G., Local active suppression and successful vaccination against spontaneous abortion in CBA/J mice, J. Reprod. Immunol. 10:79 (1987).

48. Bobe, P., Chaouat, G., Stanislawski, M., and Kiger, N., Immunogenetics of spontaneous abortion in mice. II. Anti-abortive effects are independent of systemic regulatory mechanisms, Cell Immunol. 98:477 (1987).

49. Zuckermann, F. A. and Head, J. R., Expression of MHC antigens on murine trophoblast and their modulation by interferon, J. Immunol. 137:846 (1986).

50. Clark, D. A., Host immunoregulatory mechanisms and the success of the conceptus fertilized *in vivo* and *in vitro*. In: *Early Pregnancy Failure: Mechanisms and Treatment*, R. W. Beard and F. Sharp, (eds.), Ashton-under-Lyne, U.K., Peacock Press, p. 215 (1988).

51. Clark, D. A., Brierley, J., Banwatt, D., and Chaouat, G., Hormone-induced pre-implantation Lyt-2$^+$ murine uterine suppressor cells persist after implantation and may reduce the spontaneous abortion rate in CBA/J mice, Cell. Immunol., 123:334 (1989).

52. de Fourgerolles, A. R. and Baines, M. G., Modulation of the natural killer cell activity in pregnant mice alters the spontaneous abortion rate, J. Reprod. Immunol. 11:147 (1987).

53. Clark, D. A., Head, J. R., Drake, B., Fulop, G., Brierley, J., Manuel, J., Banwatt, D., and Chaouat, G., Role of a factor related to transforming growth factor $\beta2$ in successful pregnancy. In: *Molecular Biology of the Feto-maternal Interface*, T. G. Wegmann and T. Gill, (eds.), New York, Oxford Univ. Press, (1989), *In Press*.

54. Drake, B. L. and Head, J. R., Murine trophoblast can be killed by lymphokine-activated killer cells, J. Immunol. 143:9 (1989).

55. Shimomura, K., Manda, T., Mukumoto, S., Kobayashi, K., Nakano, K., and Mori, J., Recombinant human tumor necrosis factor-a: thrombus formation is a cause of anti-tumor activity, Int. J. Cancer 41:243 (1988).

56. Bancroft, G. J., Sheehan, K. C. F., Schreiber, R. D. and Unanue, E. R., Tumor necrosis factor is involved in the T cell-independent pathway of macrophage activation in SCID mice, J. Immunol. 143:127 (1989).

57. Owen-Schaub, L. B., Gutterman, J. U., and Grimm, E. A., Synergy of tumor necrosis factor and interleukin 2 in the activation of human cytotoxic lymphocytes: effect of tumor necrosis factor a and interleukin 2 in the generation of human lymphokine-activated killer cell cytotoxicity, Cancer Res. 48:788 (1988).

58. Eades, D. K., Cornelius, P., and Pekala, P. H., Characterization of the tumor necrosis factor receptor in human placenta, Placenta 9:247 (1988).

59. Clark, D. A., Croy, B. A., Rossant, J., and Chaouat, G., Immune presensitization and local intrauterine defenses as determinants of success or failure of murine interspecies pregnancies, J.Reprod. Fert. 77:633 (1986).

60. Chaouat, G., Menu, E., Szekeres-Bartho, J., Rebut-Bonneton, C., Bustany, P., Kinsky, R., Clark, D. A., and Wegmann, T. G., Lymphokines, steroids, placental factors and trophoblast intrinsic resistance to immune cell mediated lysis are involved in pregnancy success or immunologically mediated pregnancy failure. In: *Molecular Immunology of the Feto-maternal Interface*, T. Gill and T. G. Wegmann,(eds.), New York, Oxford Univ. Press, *In Press*.

61. Chaouat, G., Menu, E., Clark, D. A., Minowsky, M., Dy, M., and Wegmann, T. G., Control of fetal survival in CBA x DBA/2 mice by lymphokine therapy, J. Reprod. Fert., 89:447 (1990).

62. Gendron, R. L. and Baines, M. G., Immunohistochemical analysis of decidual natural killer cells during spontaneous abortion in mice, Cell Immunol. 113:261 (1988).

63. Caulfield, M. J., Luce, K. J., Proffitt, M. R., and Cerny, J., Induction of idiotype-specific suppressor T cells with antigen/antibody complexes, J. Exp. Med. 157:1713 (1983).

64. Lea, R. G. and Clark, D. A., The enigma of the fetal allograft: immunosuppression versus immunostimulation. FASEB J. 3:A678 (1989).

65. Chaouat, G., Menu, E., Hofman, M., Dy, M., Minowski, M., Clark, D. A., and Wegmann, T. G., Lymphokines at the feto-maternal interface affect fetal size and survival, International Congress of Immunology (07, 1989, Berlin West), Gustav-Fischer, Stuttgart, abst #118-6, p.826, (1989).

66. Hamilton, M. S. and Hamilton, B. L., Environmental influences on immunologically associated spontaneous abortion in CBA/J mice, J. Reprod. Immunol. 11:237 (1987).

67. Michel, M., Underwood, J., Clark, D. A., Mowbray, J., and Beard, R. W., Histological and immunologic study of uterine biopsy tissue of incipiently aborting women, Amer. J. Obstet. Gynecol., 161:409 (1989)..

68. Daya, S., Clark, D. A., Delvin, C., Jarrell, J., and Chaput, A., Preliminary characterization of two types of suppressor cells in the human uterus, Fertil. Steril. 44:778 (1985).

Questions

Dr. Dey: We are doing some studies in this area, both for message and protein also, but are having some difficulty with staining with those antibodies.

Dr. Clark: Yes, you're using the TGFβ-1 marker, right? We do not find TGF-β1 suppressor factors in our supernatants. My suspicion would be that your TGFβ-1 is present in other cells, and perhaps it is not secreted. The factor which we find which seems relevant to what happens to the embryo is clearly related to another type of TGFβ, that is, the β-2 molecule.

Dr. Glasser: Have you seen any evidence for TGFβ in the metrial glands?

Dr. Clark: Metrial gland cells carry Asialo-GM1. You can see some of these cells in the labyrinth and they have the ability to kill Be6 trophoblasts. We did those experiments with Ian Stuart who is visiting from South Hampton. Whether the metrial gland is a type of LAK that is responsible for killing the embryo or whether it has a different type of effect, we don't know. We haven't yet seen cells producing the TGFβ-2 molecule in the metrial gland and there don't seem to be any suppressor factors released from the metrial triangle. The metrial triangle is outside the muscularis and our suppressor cells are lying between the muscularis and the embryo; whether suppression is present in the metrial gland area here I don't know.

13

Epilogue

The presentations of this Symposium would be incomplete without a summary and perspective as given by an experienced reproductive scientist. These perspectives were given in this Symposium by Don C. Johnson, Professor of Obstetrics and Gynecology, University of Kansas Medical Center, Kansas City. His extemporaneous comments follow.

I think I want to thank the organizing committee for this opportunity. They have been many tremendous presentations here today, it is very difficult to tie together nine hours of presentations as well as poster presentations. If I did that I would simply insult these people, and I don't want to insult them. They have done a tremendous job and we have all learned a great deal, and I think I now have a feeling for the medical students who complain about information overload. I think some of you in the audience must realize that many of these people have come here to give these presentations are actually talking to each other. You may have felt left out. I am one of these people, I don't make my living in molecular biology or biochemistry of the uterus. I only want to make use of the information these people generate for me. I want to stand back and talk to you in the audience about this, and my perspective, what I gained from this information. Some of you may come away with entirely different information about this conference.   Why are we interested in the uterus at all? We have obviously lived there at one time, and we often like to go to those places where we have been. Especially at times when you can't remember them. Let's go back and think about that. From a biological standpoint the uterus is a fantastic tissue. It is a tissue for all seasons. It produces paracrines, autocrines, endocrines. It has receptors on its cells which recognize other cells, and thus we have mechanical connections. It has intracellular and extracellular receptors. It has cells with gap junctions, so that messages can transfer from cell to cell in small molecules. Many of the graphs you saw exemplifies these things. The one part of it which makes sense is how complicated it is with all of these things. The whole program started yesterday with Dr. Bern who presented the first heresy about estrogen not being mitogenic, in spite of the fact that this has been preached at us for years. Inject estrogen, see what it does to uterine epithelium. In culture, it is inhibitory. Insulin and growth factor, EGF (epidermal growth factor), one of the first initials that we started talking about, were growth promoters *in vitro*. Next came Dr. Bigsby. He showed us the possibility of having an *in vivo/in vitro* estrogen action ratio which would be infinite. In other words, we have a DNA synthesis increase and a mitotic increase in cells which don't have estrogen receptors. Thus the ratio is infinite (zero is the denominator). Now most of us have grown up with the idea that the *in vivo/in vitro* response should be one. In this case, the estrogen receptors of the stromal cells are responsible for the agent which is giving you the estrogen action in the epithelium.

Dr. Bigsby also brought up a point which struck home to me, strain differences in response. The species and strain differences are quite important in this area and one has to recognize them. I want to digress a little bit in that area. Now most of you are aware that daughters of women who were treated with diethylstilbestrol (DES) had an increased incidence of cervical neoplasia or actual cancers of the cervix, or precancerous conditions. That particular finding stimulated new research, a lot of which was done by Dr. Bern.

Important work. The question which you need to ask the clinician is, why would anyone give a woman diethylstilbestrol? What was the point of it to begin with? The reason was that it was given because it was believed that DES would save pregnancies in women who were habitual aborters. These studies were flawed. Why? Because of the controls in the studies. Now, if you wanted to find out if giving the woman DES is going to be harmful to her offspring, who are you going to compare it to? You'll have to compare it to woman who did not have the condition for which you gave the drug. In other words, you have to take normal women, give them DES-examine their offspring-do they also have the same problem? Honestly, you would get in trouble if you tried that. However, you can do the reverse, you can look at women who are habitual aborters and who do not use diethylstilbestrol. Now there we have different type of control. When we do that the whole thing falls apart because their daughters also have a high incidence of neoplastic changes in the cervix. So it looks like DES may have gotten a bum rap. DES also got bum raps in the beef production market.

The point is that we have maybe a strain difference. How many different strains of humans do you think that there are? There must be a tremendous number of them. Does this mean then that the habitual aborter belongs to a strain of humans that now has a genetic defect which increases the expression of oncogenes which are responsible for this particular affect? The importance of that is that we should stop looking at diethylstilbestrol as the causative agent and we should start looking at something else. This is the whole point--the cell having the response is not necessarily the one we should be looking at.

We have this response in cells which do not even have the estrogen receptor. Now we can have another type of situation. We can also have estrogens which bind to receptors one way or the other and have tremendous estrogenic activity, out of proportion to their binding characteristics. I think many of you have certainly been aware of this for a long time. Estrogen is mimiced by a large variety of compounds, and I have thought about that many times and wondered why is it just estrogen? Are there any mimics for progesterone? Are there any mimics for androgen, corticosterones? Well, I do not know of them, but there are lots of mimics for estrogen. Why? Is this some sort of special situation?

I will just mention a couple more estrogen examples because here we have the same situation. We can have *in vivo/in vitro* ratios for estrogenic action which are very high. I will mention one of them, doisynolic acid. Doisynolic acid is more uterotropic than estradiol, and yet has a very weak affinity for the estradiol receptor. And since we have this mind set that the ratio must be close to one, and only those things which bind the estrogen receptor are going to give you any response, we get all mixed up with these things. We now know that is not true. We also know that some estrogen induced cells can express oncogenes, they can express growth factors, all kinds of factors. There is no reason to think that is the only compound which can induce these. In other words, you can have a chemical substance which increases the expression of *fos*, v-*mic*, or whatever. This will end up giving you an "estrogenic" response and had nothing to do with binding to the receptor at all. This research has opened up a whole new era. We do not have to be thinking only in terms of those receptors now, we can talk about secondary messengers and the other cellular molecules such as the transcription regulators. They can be turned on by another inducer which is not related to the estrogen receptor. What about other agents, the xenobiotics, the insecticides, DET, and those things which also bind to some degree to estrogen receptors. We are trying to relate biological activity to their receptor binding, and it is probably not appropriate at all. We should now be looking at this business of having other cells responsible for the estrogen action of another tissue or another cell.

In this area, you are certainly aware that EGF has been talked about a great deal. That seems to be a hormone for all seasons. It can do everything. It can get the blastocysts ready for implantation, it plays a role in implantation, and it seems to be involved in almost anything including muscle action, all kinds of activity from EGF. You will probably say, "Is that the whole story?" Obviously it is not, it is only one of them. And one of the things that scared me about Dr. Stancel's talk, is the number of growth factors we have not found yet. What do they do. How they interact with each other. That is going to be an area which is going to be enormous to unfold. On the other end of that, where I have very little information was the talk we heard this morning with Dr. Bazer. That was a beautiful summary since everything was done, you did not have to do any more. It seems so complete that there is nothing more to do there. Which, of course, could not be farther from the truth. There was a lot of data there and it is a pretty story, but there are a lot of question marks which will give them a job for a long time to come. And this is one of the things that I suppose that a conference like this does. It makes you think that we have come a long way and we have a tremendous amount of information here, and we should pat ourselves on the back. Well, perhaps so, but on the other hand, it is really scary and we have an awful lot of questions that we have not answered and we have a long way to go.

Now where are we going to go from here? Someone has already mentioned that if we had this conference next year we would learn a great deal more. Well, maybe next year is a little bit too soon. I think we will need to wait a little bit longer than that before we are going to get very far. But certainly we can see down the future what is going to happen, or at least, what we think is going to happen. We certainly have not conquered the world population problem by any means. And the politicians will sooner or later will come to roost on it again, that we really ought to do something about that.

In the last forty years, we have dwelt upon the pituitary and ovary as places for fertility control, and to a much lesser extent, the testis. We know that is because when we look at the majority of this audience it is male, and so that we have not nearly concentrated as much time on the males as the females.

We can also see from what has been presented yesterday and today, that we are coming into the age of the uterus. Future experiments in fertility control, are very likely to be in the area of the uterus. So what we can hope for is that we will have an increase in funding, and I think all of us would like to see something there because these experiments are going to be expensive, and in a few years coming down the road, this area is going to expand fantastically, and fertility control mechanisms very likely will narrow down to the uterus.

The control of implantation is something which we have heard a great deal about, and is an area in which there is really a great deal of mystery yet, but we had some encouraging reports. Dr. Glasser's model system of polarity suggests we may now have a closer handle on implantation, which will also be very valuable for the fertility people who want to increase fertility and not decrease it. I think the future of this system is very bright, and I hope we can have a conference, perhaps, in five years, and really open up great deal more of information. Maybe we will have learned more by then about the how the cytokines fit into this thing as well as the growth factors.

Poster Presentation Abstracts

Induction of mRNA for CBG during pregnancy and pseudopregnancy of the hamster

Lin GX, Selcer KW, Beale EG
Department of Cell Biology and Anatomy, Texas Tech University Health Sciences Center, Lubbock, TX

We have previously presented evidence for a decidua-hepatic endocrine axis in which the decidualized uterus signals the liver to produce certain pregnancy-associated serum proteins. We have shown that: 1) serum levels of corticosteroid-binding globulin (CBG) increase in the pregnant and pseudopregnant hamster, and this increase is related to the presence of decidual tissue; 2) hepatocytes from the pregnant hamster produce substantially more CBG than those from the nonpregnant hamster; and, 3) removal of the decidualized uterus interrupts the CBG response.

The purpose of the present study was to measure changes in levels of CBG-mRNA in the liver and various nonhepatic tissues during pregnancy and pseudopregnancy of the hamster. A cRNA was prepared from rat cDNA for CBG (obtained from G. Hammond) and used to evaluate the RNA extracted from the various tissues using solution hybridization assays and Northern blot procedures. Northern blot analysis of hamster and rat liver RNA revealed that the rat probe hybridized with hamster liver mRNA and pregnant liver contained more mRNA than nonpregnant liver. The relative amount of mRNA was measured by solution hybridization assay under conditions where the RNA was varied and ^{32}p-cRNA was held constant. The linear portion of the hybridization curve was resolved for each RNA preparation and the relative difference in mRNA content was determined by slope-ratio analysis. Liver RNA from late pregnant hamster (day 14) contained 39-fold more CBG-mRNA than nonpregnant hamster liver. When RNA from other tissues (kidney, spleen, small intestine, decidual tissue) was assayed, a small but significant signal was detected by solution hybridization. However, Northern blot analysis of the RNA from nonhepatic tissues showed that the small amount of hybridizable sequences did not exist as mature mRNA and may represent nuclear precursor or another form of RNA. A time-course of changes in hepatic mRNA during pregnancy revealed a significant increase in CBG mRNA by day 4 of pregnancy. CBG-mRNA levels increased to a peak during late pregnancy (days 12-15) and decreased by day 16 before parturition. A time-course analysis during pseudopregnancy (days 4-9) showed an increase in CBG-mRNA by day 5, a peak on days 6 and 7, and a decrease on days 8 and 9.

This reveals that hepatic CBG-mRNA is induced during decidualization. Changes in serum CBG (as measured by ^{3}H-cortisol binding assay) closely paralleled those of hepatic CBG-mRNA. The positive correlation between hepatic CBG-mRNA levels and serum CBG suggests that regulation of serum CBG in the pregnant and the pseudopregnant hamster occurs at the level of hepatic gene transcription.

This work was supported by National Institutes of Health grants kHD18712,HD07271 and GM39895.

Suppression of interleukin-2 utilization by hydatidiform mole trophoblast extracts is neutralized by pre-incubation with monoclonal α-interferon antibody

Bennett WA, Brackin MN, Cowan BD
Department of Obstetrics and Gynecology, University of Mississippi Medical Center
Jackson, MS

In domestic animals (sheep, cattle, pigs), α-interferon-like proteins of trophoblast origin have been implicated as embryonic signals involved in the maternal recognition of pregnancy (Roberts, 1989). Trophoblast extracts (HME) from human hydatidiform molar pregnancies contain macromolecule(s) which suppress T cell proliferation in response to mitogen (Cowan et al., 1989) or interleukin-2 (Bennett et al., 1988). To determine if this activity was due to an α-interferon-like factor, HME was preincubated (5% CO_2, 95% air) for 1 hour at 37° C with anti-interferon-α monoclonal antibody (anti-IFN α-Mab) from mouse ascites (Boehringer-Mannheim) prior to addition to a human interleukin-2 (IL-2) utilization assay. For this assay, PHA-treated human T lymphocytes (PHA-blasts) were stimulated with maximal concentrations (10 U/well or 50 U/ml) of human recombinant IL-2 (ICN).

Addition of 500 μg of HME significantly ($p < 0.05$) suppressed PHA-blast proliferation (44.6% of controls) in response to 10 U of IL-2. The preincubation with either 200 U or 500 U of anti-IFNα MAb significantly ($p < 0.05$) reduced the suppressive effect of HME (106.4% and 78.8% of controls, respectively). No effect was observed when 20 U of α-IFN Ab was added to the molar extract (46.1% of controls). The α-IFN Ab did not affect PHA-blast proliferation in the absence of exogenous IL-2 at any of the concentrations tested. HME suppressed ($p < 0.05$) proliferation of the PHA-blasts in the absence of IL-2 (55.0% of controls), and this suppression was not overcome with the addition of anti-IFNα-MAb at the concentrations used in the IL-2 stimulation studies.

These results suggest that hydatidiform mole trophoblast contains an α-interferon-like factor capable of suppressing Il-2 utilization by activated T lymphocytes.

This project was supported by grant #2 807 RR05386 awarded by the Biomedical Research Support Grant Program, Division of Research Resources, National Institutes of Health and the Vicksburg Hospital Foundation.

Hormone-dependent uterine adenocarcinoma following developmental treatment with estrogen

Newbold RR, Bullock BC, Trasti LD, McLachlan JA
Developmental Endocrinology and Pharmacology Section, Laboratory of Reproductive and Developmental Toxicology, Division of Intramural Research, National Institute of Environmental Health Sciences, National Institutes of Health, Research Triangle Park, NC

Although estrogens are associated with neoplasia in target tissues including cervix, uterus and breast, the mechanism(s) underlying this association are still not clear.

To develop a model to study target organ specific hormonal carcinogenesis, outbred female mice were treated with diethylstilbestrol (DES) on day 1-5 of neonatal life and sacrificed from 1 to 18 months of age. Uterine adenocarcinoma was observed in a time and dose related manner after DES treatment; at 18 months of age, neoplastic lesions were seen in 90% of the mice exposed neonatally to the highest DES dose (2 μg/pup/day) while no uterine tumors were seen in the corresponding control mice. These DES-induced uterine tumors were estrogen dependent. When mice with established uterine tumors were ovariectomized, the lesions regressed; estrogen treatment reestablished the lesion's growth. Also, ovariectomizing neonatal DES-treated mice before puberty prevented uterine lesions from occurring later in life. As a marker for neoplasia, uterine cancers were transplanted as tissue fragments and carried as serial transplants in nude mice. The transplanted tissue retained some differentiated uterine functions and also required estrogen supplementation for maintenance. In addition, several cell lines were established and characterized from the DES-induced uterine tumors. Additional studies compared neonatal treatment of mice with various DES analogs (hexestrol, dienestrol, tetrafluroDES) and steroidal estrogens. There was an apparent correlation of estrogenicity and uterine carcinogenicity in neonatal life. All compounds except estradiol were capable of inducing uterine adenocarcinoma by 12 months of age. Higher doses of estradiol were also able to induce uterine tumors by the incidence was lower as compared to the number of lesions induced by DES. These experiments provide the basis for subsequent studies in the mechanisms of hormonal carcinogenesis.

Mouse uterine cell differentiation and estrogen responsiveness *in vitro*

Burroughs CD, Ross KA, Ignar DM, Nelson KG, Takahashi T, Korach KS, McLachlan JA
Laboratory of Reproductive and Developmental Toxicology, National Institutes of Environmental Health Sciences, Research Triangle Park, NC

Although estrogens are potent stimulants of uterine cell proliferation *in vivo*, there has been no clear demonstration of estrogen induced proliferation of normal uterine cells grown as monolayer culture *in vitro*. The present studies were conducted to determine whether appropriate differentiation may be necessary for the estrogen responsiveness of two uterine cell types (stroma and epithelium) separately maintained *in vitro*. Uterine epithelial cells were isolated from immature female CD-1 mice (17 days old) by trypsinization and Percoll density gradient centrifugation and cultured on a specially prepared phenol red free biomatrix (Matrigel^R- Collaborative Research). Stromal cells were also isolated from immature mouse uteri and cultured on plastic. Both uterine cell types were maintained in a 1:1 mixture of Hams-F12 and Dulbeccos Modified Eagles media supplemented with $CaCl_2$ (0.1 mM), bovine serum albumin (0.1%), amphotericin B (2.5 μg/ml), insulin (10μg/ml), and transferrin (10 μg/ml). In some cases epidermal growth factor (EFG; 10 ng/ml) and/or 17-β-estradiol (E2; 10^{9}M) was added.

Initially (within 1-2 days) the epithelial cells on Matrigel form a monolayer; by day 8 of culture the cells from three dimensional, tube-like structures. Even though these uterine epithelial cells exhibited a more differentiated morphology, estrogen did not stimulate growth. However, E2 treatment of cultured uterine stromal cells consistently resulted in a decreased rate of proliferation. The presence of EGF did not influence either the epithelial or stromal cell response to estrogen. Preliminary results, using affinity labeling and Western Blot analysis, indicate that uterine epithelial cells have lower estrogen receptor (ER) levels than stromal cells after 8 days of culture, but equivalent levels at the beginning of culture. Immunohistochemical techniques are being used to localize both the ER and progesterone receptor (PGR) in these cultures. In addition to evaluating the growth response of these cultures to estrogen, we are determining whether estrogen can induce specific genes such as PGR and lactotransferrin, both of which are estrogen inducible *in vivo*. This cell culture system will aid in the study of the relationship of estrogen associated differentiation and proliferation in the two uterine cell types.

Purification and growth characteristics of bovine uterine epithelial and stroma cells

Helmer SD, Zavy MT, Geisert RD
USDA, ARS, Forage and Livestock Research Laboratory, El Reno, OK and OAES, Stillwater, OK

The purpose of this study was to obtain purified populations of bovine uterine epithelial and stroma (ST) cells. Reproductive tracts were recovered from 7 Hereford cows in Phase I and II, at day 5 of the estrous cycle. Uterine horns were filled with Pancreatin-dispase and incubated for 1.5 h while increasing water bath temperature from 4 to 37° C. Surface epithelial rafts were recovered from the enzyme wash and one to two washes with Ca, Mg-free Hank's (CMFH) and glands from subsequent washes. Cellular rafts and glands were then isolated on 20 μm screens, recovered and dissociated in CMFH by mechanical agitation. Stromal cells were obtained from CMFH washes after an additional incubation with PBS-dispase. Epithelial cells were plated at 37,500 and 62,500 cells/cm^2 in phase I and II, respectively. Stroma cells were plated at 2,500 cells/cm^2 in both phases. Cell purity was assessed visually and by specific cytoskeletal staining of the intermediate filaments cytokeratin (epithelium) and vimentin (ST). Growth characteristics at various seeding densities was evaluated. Epithelia seeded between 25,000 and 250,000 cells/cm^2 reached confluence in approx 15 and 9 days (surface epithelium, SE) and 17 and 10 days (glandular epithelium, GE), respectively. Stroma were seeded at between 2,500 and 250,000 cells/cm^2 which attained confluence in approx 9 and 1-2 days, respectively. Cells were grown in culture flasks and protein secretory profiles of culture supernatants analyzed by 2-D SDS-PAGE and, silver stain procedures. Some proteins were common to all cell types compared to control media while more proteins were found in supernatants from GE cells (M$_r$ approx 28,000, pI approx 6.8-7.8 and M$_r$ approx 66,000 and pI approx 4.0). Surface epithelial and ST cells were also grown on several matrices. Matrices (plastic, laminin, fibronectin, type IV collagen, type I collagen and matrigel) were applied to culture wells at 1.375 μg/cm^2 in 24 well plates in both phases and 2.15 and 1.375 μg/cm^2 in 96 well plates in Phase I and II, respectively. Growth was evaluated visually and by measuring cellular protein, DNA content, cell number and incorporation of ^{3}H-thymidine. Cells were harvested on day 1, 2, 4, 8 of incubation in Phase I and on day 3, 6, 9, and 12 (ST) and 3, 6, 9 and 15 (SE) in Phase II. Cells from 12 wells per day/matrix in Phase I and 6 wells per day/matrix in Phase II were harvested, concentrated and aliquoted. Epithelial cells generally did not reach confluence in Phase I due to a low seeding density. As a result of this, no significant results were noted. Cells tended to grow better on plastic and type IV collagen while doing poorly on matrigel. After increasing seeding density and incubation interval SE cells reached confluence in Phase II. Significantly more DNA was contained in cells grown on plastic and type IV collagen than in cells grown on other matrices. There were no significant effects due to matrix for cell number or protein content though cells tended to perform better on plastic and collagen with poor performance on laminin and matrigel. Stroma generally grew to confluence in Phase I. Cells grown on matrigel had more protein (p < 0.05) compared to cells grown on other matrices. Differences in protein and thymidine incorporation in ST cells in Phase I were not significant, but results indicated that cells performed well on matrigel and laminin while performing poorly on fibronectin. There were no significant treatment effects seen in Phase II for ST cells, however, cells performed best on plastic while performing poorly on fibronectin and matrigel. Epithelial and ST growth performance on the matrices tested was variable with SE generally performing well on plastic and collagen and poorly on matrigel. Whereas, ST performed well on matrigel and laminin in Phase I and plastic and collagen in Phase II while doing poorly on fibronectin in both cases. These results indicate that several matrices are adequate to support growth of bovine SE and stroma cells.

Role of epidermal growth factor on implantation in the mouse

Gupta A, Dey SK
Department of Obstetrics and Gynecology and Physiology, University of Kansas
Medical Center, Kansas City, KS

Recently we have observed that estrogen-induced initiation of implantation in a progesterone (P4)-primed uterus is mediated via prostaglandin E_2 (PGE_2) as a component of Phase I of estrogen action (Endocrinology 124:546, 1989). However, it is not yet defined how this response is triggered by estrogen. A recent report indicates the epidermal growth factor (EGF) stimulates synthesis of cyclooxygenase in smooth muscle cells in culture (FASEB J 2:2613, 1988). Furthermore, our recent study has established that EGF gene is expressed and EGF protein accumulates in the mouse uterus during the preimplantation period under the influence of estrogen (J Cell Biochem, in press).

These observations suggest that one of the functions of preimplantation ovarian estrogen secretion in a P_4-dominated mouse uterus prior to implantation (J Endocrinol 62:101, 1974) could be to stimulate uterine synthesis and/or release of EGF which then stimulates the synthesis and/or release of PGs in the uterus and/or embryo and initiates the process of implantation in an autocrine/paracrine fashion. We used estriol (E3) because this estrogen, when given as a single injection, elicits primarily Phase I responses and initiates implantation in a P_4-primed uterus. CD-1 female mice (48 days old) were ovariectomized on day 4 of pregnancy (day 1 = vaginal plug) and injected with P_4 (2 mg/0.1 ml sesame oil/mouse, s.c.) for 4 days to induce delayed implantation. Implantation in the mouse occurs on the evening of day 4. On the last day of P_4 treatment (i.e., 4 days of delay), they were given a single injection of indomethacin (100 or 250 μg/0.1 ml oil/mouse, s.c.) 30 min prior to an injection of E3 (100 ng/0.1 ml oil/mouse, s.c.) or the same dose of E3 plus a single injection of various doses of EGF (100 ng, 250 ng, 500 ng and 5 μg/0.1 ml saline/mouse, i.p.). The initiation of implantation was examined 24 h later by an intravenous injection of 0.1 ml of a 0.1% Chicago Blue B solution in 0.15 M NaCl. The discrete blue bands along the uterus indicated implantation sites. While indomethacin, an inhibitor of cyclooxygenase, interfered with E3-inducible implantation in 70% (14/20) of the animals, a co-injection of EGF (250 ng-5 μg) with E3 completely reversed the indomethacin-induced inhibition of implantation in all animals (14/14 with 4-5 animals per treatment group). However, EGF at 100 ng was not effective. These results suggest that estrogen apparently stimulates the uterine synthesis and/or release of EGF which in turn induces the synthesis/release of uterine and/or embryonic PGs that initiates the process of implantation. However, PGE_2, EGF, or a combination of PGE_2 and EGF failed to initiate implantation in the absence of E3. These later findings suggest that while PGE_2 and EGF are involved, they are not the sole mediators of implantation. This is not surprising because the process of implantation is a complex interaction between the uterine and embryonic cells which respond uniquely to steroid hormones. We have previously observed that both the uterus and the blastocyst must be exposed to estrogen for successful implantation (Life Sci 27:2381, 1980). Thus, estrogen appears to operate in this process via separate mechanisms that involve preparation of the uterus and activation of the blastocyst. The failure of PGE_2 and EGF to trigger implantation in the absence of E3 is perhaps due to their lack of influence on one of these sites of estrogen action. In other words, these mediators may be functional in the uterus, but may be unable to activate the blastocyst or vice-versa. Further investigation will be required to resolve this issue.

Cytokine regulation of murine decidual metallothionein gene expression

McMaster MT, De SK, Dey SK, Andrews GK
Department of Biochemistry and Molecular Biology, The University of Kansas Medical Center, Kansas City, KS

Metallothionein (MT) mRNAs are present at high levels in decidua on days 5-10 of pregnancy (D1 = vaginal plug). Expression of the MT genes also occurs in experimentally induced deciduomata which suggests that it is independent of the embryo. In many tissues, metal ions (Zn), glucocorticoids, or bacterial lipopolysaccharide-endotoxin (LPS) induced cytokines are the most potent inducers of MT mRNA.

In order to examine the mechanisms of regulation of decidual MT gene expression, the competence of the D4 pregnant uterus to respond to these agents was determined. MT mRNA levels in D8 decidua are much greater than those in the maternal liver which suggests a local effect on MT genes in decidua. Injection of Zn resulted in only a slight increase in MT mRNA in the D4 uterus, whereas liver MT mRNA levels were maximally stimulated. This establishes that the D4 uterus is not highly responsive to Zn, and suggests that systemic changes in metal ion concentrations do not account for elevated decidual MT mRNA levels. Adrenalectomy on D4 did not effect MT mRNA levels in decidua on D8, indicating that glucocorticoids do not play a significant role in decidual MT expression. Furthermore, treatment of ovariectomized mice with progesterone and/or estrogen had little effect on MT mRNA levels in the uterus. Injection of LPS or human recombinant interleukin-1 (IL-1α) rapidly elevated MT mRNA levels several-fold in the D4 uterus. Following injection of LPS or IL-1α, rapid induction of mRNAs for a variety of cytokines (i.e. IL-1α, IL-1β and tumor necrosis factor-α (TNF-α)) occurred in the D4 uterus. These results establish that exogenous cytokines can enhance MT gene expression in the uterus, and that several cytokine genes in this organ can be up-regulated. Northern blot analysis demonstrated the presence of IL-1α, IL-1β and TNF-α mRNAs, and immunocytochemistry detected IL-1α and TNF-α in the untreated decidua.

These results lead us to hypothesize that expression of MT genes in decidua is regulated in an autocrine/paracrine manner by cytokines which are produced locally in response to the pro-inflammatory process of implantation and decidualization.

Cellular and molecular characterization of the post-mating uterine inflammatory response in the mouse

Sanford TH[1], De M[1], Andrews GA[2], Wood GW[1]
Departments of Pathology and Oncology[1] and Biochemistry and Molecular Biology[2]
University of Kansas Medical Center, Kansas City, KS

Early morphologic studies of the progestational uterus established that mating is followed by an inflammatory response to sperm and semen which is characterized by an early influx of granulocytes followed by a mononuclear infiltrate which abates prior to implantation. The present study was designed to assess progestational changes in bone marrow-derived cells both numerically and functionally using immunological and molecular methodology. Immunohistochemical analysis of uterine tissues with anti-macrophage (F4/80) and anti-common leukocyte antigen (M1/9.3.4.HL.2) antibodies revealed a massive accumulation of macrophages in the subepithelial stroma on day 1. The response was reduced on day 2 and, by day 3, macrophage numbers and distribution had returned to a level comparable to diestrus. On day 4, macrophages again were concentrated in subepithelial stroma, but no quantitative changes were observed. Quantitative immunocytochemical analysis of uterine cell suspensions confirmed the tissue results; large numbers of lymphocytes, macrophages and granulocytes were present in suspensions on day 1 and 2, but on days 3 and 4 the common leukocyte antigen positive cells were primarily macrophages. Bioassays of the soluble fraction of uterine tissue homogenates revealed an association between the inflammatory response and production of colony stimulating factors for macrophages and mast cells on day 1 which was reduced on day 2, undetectable on day 3 and elevated again on day 4. There was no evidence for formation of myeloid colonies, indicating that granulocyte colony stimulating factor production was low or absent during days 1-4. Northern blot analysis of uterine poly A RNA revealed a relatively high level of CSF-1 mRNA on day 1 which was slightly decreased on days 2-4. IL-3 mRNA was detectable on days 1, 2 and 4 but not day 3. GM-CSF mRNA was detectable only on day 1. These data demonstrated a quantitative relationship between the cellular infiltrate and local production of cytokines which cause accumulation of bone marrow derived cells. To analyze macrophage function during the same time period, bioassays for the monokines, IL-1 and TNFα, were performed on uterine tissue supernatants. A significant amount of TNFα was detectable, but no quantitative changes were observed between days 1 and 4. In sharp contrast, IL-1 was very high on day 1, low on day 2 and very high again on days 3 and 4. The bioassay results were parallel by results obtained from Northern blot analyses of uterine poly A RNA for the macrophage gene products, IL-1α, IL-1β, IL-6 and TNFα. The accumulated data demonstrated that introduction of semen and sperm to the receptive uterus induces an inflammatory response which is indistinguishable from classical inflammatory responses to, for example, bacteria on both a cellular and a molecular level. The data also demonstrated that significant alterations in macrophage numbers and function occur during the preimplantation period, suggesting that they and their products play an important role in preparing the uterus for implantation.

Relationship between uterine cytokine production and macrophage distribution during murine pregnancy

De M, Sanford T, Choudhuri R, Wood GW
Department of Pathology and Oncology, University of Kansas Medical Center, Kansas City, KS

The purpose of this study was to quantitate macrophage numbers and function in the murine uterus between implantation and parturition. A monoclonal antibody specific for mature macrophages (F4/80) was employed in quantitative and distributional immunocytochemical analysis of tissues and cell suspensions. The results for the preimplantation period are reported elsewhere (See Sanford, *et al.*, this meeting). On day 4, macrophages were concentrated in the subepithelial endometrium, a distribution which was maintained through day 5. The number of macrophages increased in the endometrium between days 4 and 5, and on day 5 macrophages were observed in association with the luminal epithelium at the site of blastocyst attachment. With the development of the primary decidua in the antimesometrial uterus on day 6, macrophages were displaced toward the periphery of the uterus. Macrophage concentration remained high in the interimplantation zones. Beginning on day 6, cells expressing common leukocyte antigen (M1/9.3.4.HL.2) were observed accumulating in the mesometrial uterus around remaining luminal epithelium. Those cells continued to increase in number throughout pregnancy and were morphologically and immunohistochemically indistinguishable from cells comprising the decidua basalis and the metrial gland. Those cells also expressed low levels of macrophage antigen.

To investigate possible mechanisms responsible for accumulation of such large numbers of bone-marrow derived cells, colony stimulating factor activity was quantitated by bioassay in supernatants of uterine tissue homogenates. No granulocyte colony stimulating activity was present at any time, but high levels of mast cell and macrophage colony stimulating activity were evident on day 4, then again on days 7 through 18. That bioactivity was reflected in increasing levels of CSF-1 mRNA detected by Northern blot analysis of days 4-18 uterine RNA. To assess functional activity of uterine macrophages, IL-1 and TNFα, monokines with a wide range of biological activities, were quantitated. IL-1 bioactivity (specific antibody inhibitable activity in a thymocyte proliferation assay) exhibited a major peak on day 4, was low on days 5-8 and elevated from days 9 to 18. IL-1α, but not IL-1β, mRNA levels were strikingly similar to the bioassay results. In contrast, TNFα bioactivity (specific antibody inhibitable L929 fibroblast cytotoxicity) was significant, but relatively constant until increases were observed on days 15 and 16 and very high levels were observed on days 17 and 18. TNFα mRNA levels were constant throughout the post-implantation period. Two major conclusions can be derived from these data: 1) there is a direct relationship between CSF-1 production in the uterus and macrophage numbers and distribution; and 2) during three important periods of fetal development, macrophage function, assessed by IL-1 production, is markedly elevated.

Products of LPS-activated macrophages (TNF-α, TGF-β) but not LPS alter DNA synthesis by LPS receptor-bearing rat trophoblast cells

Hunt JS, Soares MJ, Morrison DC
Departments of Pathology, Physiology and Microbiology, University of Kansas Medical Center, Kansas City, KS

Pregnancy losses from gram negative bacterial infections could be caused by direct effects of lipopolysaccharide (LPS) on placental cells, or indirectly via LPS activation of macrophages in the uteroplacental unit. To evaluate these alternatives, LPS, LPS-activated peritoneal cells (PC), conditioned medium from LPS-activated PC, and some purified and recombinant molecules known to be secreted by activated macrophages were tested for their abilities to modify DNA synthesis by three rat trophoblast cell lines. Although LPS receptors were demonstrated on trophoblast cells, LPS alone had no effect on the ability of trophoblast cells to synthesize DNA. Both LPS-stimulated PC and conditioned media from LPS-activated PC were highly inhibitory to trophoblast cell DNA synthesis. When specific molecules likely to be components of those media were tested, IL-1 was found to have a modest but reproducible stimulatory effect and PGE_2 did not change trophoblast cell incorporation of ^3H-thymidine. In contrast, trophoblast cell DNA synthesis was markedly inhibited in a dose-dependent manner by both TNF-α and TGF-β1. No differences in the sensitivity of trophoblast cells from outbred and inbred rats were observed. The results suggest that in cases of infection by gram negative bacteria, LPS may have an adverse effect on pregnancy by stimulating resident macrophages to generate and release molecules that are inhibitory to trophoblast cell DNA synthesis.

Supported in part by the March of Dimes Foundation for Birth Defects and the Wesley Foundation.

Progestin and glucocorticoid stimulation of synthesis of a secretory protein produced by rabbit stromal cells in culture

Everett LM, Bigsby RM
Department of Obstetrics and Gynecology, Indiana University, Indianapolis, IN

Endometrial stromal cells from ovariectomized rabbits were cultured in Ham's F12/DME plus BSA, insulin and antibiotics. The synthesis and secretion of a protein of approximately 42 kD was studied using ^{35}S-methionine labeling, SDS-PAGE of medium products and densitometric analysis of resultant fluorograms.

Synthesis of the protein was enhanced approximately 1.5-2.0 fold by treating cultures with 10^{-7} M progesterone (P), deoxycorticosterone (DOC), or dexamethasone (DEX). The response was dose dependent over the range of 10^{-10}-10^{-6} M P and cells remained responsive to P stimulation for 72 hours. When P was continuously present in the medium, however, enhancement of this protein was only apparent for 48 hours; after 72 hours there was evidence of an increase in the amount of a protein of approximately 53 kD. Addition of estradiol did not increase the number of the 42 kD protein present in the medium. There was no modification of the P response either by priming the cells with estradiol (10^{-9} M) for 24 hours prior to adding P or by addition of estradiol simultaneously with P. The P antagonists ZK98734 and ZK98299 (Schering AG) blocked stimulation of the protein by both P and DOC but appeared to have only a partial inhibitory effect on DEX stimulation. Thus, the 42 kD protein may represent a gene product whose transcription is enhanced by both progestins and glucocorticoids.

Supported by grants from the Center for Alternatives to Animal Testing and National Institutes of Health grant, HD23244.

Effects of neonatal diethylstilbestrol (DES) exposure on the growth of mouse vaginal epithelial cells in serum-free collagen gel culture

Uchima F-DA, Iguchi T, Bern HA
Department of Integrative Biology and Cancer Research Laboratory, University of California at Berkeley, Berkeley, CA

Vaginal epithelial cells were isolated 10-11 days after ovariectomy of *ca* 40 day-old BALBc/cCrgl mice treated with sesame oil or 1.0 μg DES for the first 5 days after birth, and grown in primary culture using a collagen gel matrix (CGM) and 20 mM HEPES-buffered, serum-free complete (SFc) medium (Dulbecco's MEM/Ham's F-12 medium, 1:1, supplemented with epidermal growth factor (EGF), insulin, cholera toxin, transferrin and bovine serum albumin (BSA, fraction V) as in Iguchi *et al.*, Proc Natl Acad Sci 80:3743, 1983). Three-dimensional colonies of both control and DES-exposed vaginal cells developed in CGM. Initial rates of proliferation of DES-exposed vaginal cells were lower than in controls. Control vaginal cells showed an 8-fold increase; DES-exposed vaginal cells showed a 5-fold increase in cell number at day 10 in the time study. The differential effects of individual deletion of constituents from the SFc medium in the growth of vaginal cells from control and DES-exposed mice were determined. During the 9-day culture period, deletion of BSA, insulin, or EGF lowered the proliferation of control vaginal cells, whereas the deletion of insulin or EGF lowered the proliferation of DES-exposed vaginal cells. Estradiol-17β (E2, 0.18 fM to 18 nM) did not stimulate growth of vaginal cells from either control or DES-exposed mice; instead, E2 generally slowed growth (see Tsai *et al.*, this Symposium). If EGF concentration is decreased from the usual 10 ng/ml level in SFc medium, there is a corresponding dose-related (0.1-10 ng/ml) decrease in growth of vaginal cells from both control and DES-exposed mice. Thus, neonatal DES exposure results in alterations in vaginal epithelial cells as indicated by decreased proliferation and by decreased dependence on a factor (BSA) present in the SFc medium. We are presently examining the dose-related responses to other components of the SFc medium.

We acknowledge the assistance of KT MIlls and S Pattamakom. This work was supported by National Institutes of Health grant CA-05388.

Estrogen-independent proliferation and differentiation of prepubertal mouse vaginal epithelial cells in primary culture

Tsai P-S, Hamamoto ST, Uchima F-DA, Bern HA
Department of Integrative Biology and Cancer Research Laboratory, University of California at Berkeley, Berkeley, CA

Estrogen-independent proliferation and differentiation of prepubertal mouse vaginal epithelial cells in serum-free primary cultures were examined. Vaginal epithelial cells were isolated from *ca* 21-day-old female BALB/cCRGL mice according to a method modified from Iguchi *et al.* (Proc Natl Acad Sci 80:3743, 1983). At the age of 21 days, vaginal epithelium consisted of 2-4 layers of cuboidal cells and a superficial layer of tall mucified cells. Isolated cell clumps were cultured in collagen gel matrix (CGM) in a serum-free medium (SF_{20}) consisted of DMEM:Ham's F12 (1 vol:1 vol) buffered with 20 mM HEPES and supplemented with insulin, transferrin, mouse epidermal growth factor, and BSA (fraction V). Vaginal epithelial colonies cultured for 2 days were small and consisted of 1-2 layers of cuboidal cells and a lumen filled with cellular debris and PAS-positive materials. By day 6 of culture, average colony size increased approximately 10-fold, and colonies contained stratified squamous epithelium with a superficial layer of mucified cells around the lumen. By day 8 of culture, keratin formation was observed and the mucified layer was exfoliated into the lumen. Electron microscopy confirms differentiative changes observed by histological study and shows that at day 4 of culture, three types of cells were present in a single colony: 1) glandular epithelial cells with surface microvilli, apical secretory vesicles, characteristic tight junctions and desmosomes; 2) squamous cells rich in cytoplasmic tonofilaments; and, 3) low cuboidal basal cells with small, densely-stained nuclei. At day 8 of culture, the secretory cells were not evident, and squamous cells became more numerous, showing signs of terminal differentiation. Vaginal epithelial cells proliferated in SF_{20} without estrogen addition and increased 6-fold in cell number at day 10 of culture. Addition of 17β-estradiol reduced cellular proliferation by *ca* 30-50%.

Our laboratory has already demonstrated that this 17β-estradiol-induced growth retardation can be reversed by keoxifene, an antiestrogen (Tsai *et al.*, Proc AACR 30:298, 1989). Other estrane derivatives (17α-estradiol and estriol) at equimolar concentrations also reduce cellular proliferation, but to a less extent than 17β-estradiol. Thus, prepubertal mouse vaginal epithelial cells establish polarity in CGM along with exhibiting characteristics of epithelial cells. Also, spontaneous proliferation and differentiation of these cells occur *in vitro* without estrogen in the medium, and the addition of various estrane-derivatives reduces this proliferation.

We acknowledge the assistance of S Pattamakom. This work was supported by National Institutes of Health grant CA-05388 and CA-09041.

Androgen receptors in the rhesus monkey endometrium

Brenner RM and West NB
Division of Reproductive Biology and Behavior, Oregon Regional Primate Research
Center, Beaverton, OR

Monoclonal antibodies against the human androgen receptor have recently been prepared in Dr. Shutsung Liao's laboratory, University of Chicago. We have used these new reagents to evaluate the cellular localization and hormonal regulation of androgen receptors in the uterus of the rhesus monkey. All of the monoclonal antibodies we have tried, courtesy of Dr. Liao (specifically AN1-15, AN1-7 and AN1-6) recognize the monkey androgen receptor in both immunocytochemical assays and sucrose density gradient analyses. Levels of androgen receptor are low in spayed animals, elevated in estrogenized ones and significantly lowered by sequential progestin treatment. Immunocytochemical studies show that all zones of the endometrium are positive for androgen receptor, that epithelial and stromal cells both contain receptor, and that progestin treatment suppresses androgen receptor more dramatically in stromal than epithelial cells. All specific staining is localized within cell nuclei regardless of hormonal treatment. Like other members of the steroid receptor family, the androgen receptor in uterine cells is a nuclear protein whose levels can be influenced by estrogens and progestins. Androgens may play a role in endometrial hyperplasia and the development of adenocarcinoma. These new antibodies will greatly facilitate analysis of the role of androgens in uterine growth.

Progesterone not interferon α-2 suppresses endometrial PG synthesis in early human pregnancy

Smith SK[1], Mitchell SM[1], Kelly RW[2]
Department of Obstetrics and Gynaecology, University of Cambridge Rosie Maternity Hospital, Hills Road, Cambridge[1], and MRC Reproductive Biology Unit, 37 Chalmers Street, Edinburgh, UK[2]

It has been assumed in women that the reduced synthesis of PGs by early human decidua is the consequence of the continued secretion of progesterone from the corpus luteum. Recent evidence suggests that species with epithelio-chorial placentation secrete a trophoblastic protein which also suppresses PG synthesis. Theses proteins haver partial sequence homology with human interferon α-2 which suppresses PG synthesis from sheep endometrium. The aim of these studies was to investigate the mechanism of progesterone induced inhibition of PG release from human decidua by using the new anti-progestins RU 486 and ZK 98734 and to investigate the effect of interferon α-2 on PG synthesis from human endometrium.

Endometrium and decidua were obtained at operations performed for benign conditions. The tissue was partially digested with collagenase (1 mg/ml) and DNase (0.2 mg/ml) and enriched glandular preparations prepared by retaining the glands on filters. Incubations were undertaken in serum-free medium for 24 h to determine the effect of RU 486 and ZK 98734 on PG synthesis and the action of interferon α-2 on PG synthesis was investigated daily over a total of four days in culture.

The anti-progestins RU 486 and ZK 98734 increased PG synthesis from decidual glands (Smith and Kelly, 1987) suggesting that PG synthesis in early human decidua is suppressed by progesterone and that this mechanism involves binding of progesterone to its specific nuclear receptor. This increase in PG release was inhibited by actinomycin (1,100,500 and 1,000 nmol) and verapamil (5 and 10 μmol) indicating the need for new protein synthesis and a requirement for extracellular calcium. Interferon α-2 (5, 50, 500 U/ml) did not suppress PG release from enriched preparations of glands from proliferative or secretory endometrium maintained for four days in the presence of estradiol-17β (100 nmol) and did not inhibit the rise of PG release induced by exogenous AA.

Previous animal studies have usually used whole endometrium or total cellular preparations of endometrium to investigate the early pregnancy suppression of PG synthesis. Our findings in the human have shown that the glandular cells are the principal source of PG synthesis and it is from these cells that progesterone probably inhibits PG synthesis from glandular cells of human decidua by binding to its nuclear receptor and altering genomic events and that interferon α-2 does not affect PG release from glandular cells of human endometrium.

Steady state levels of epidermal growth factor messenger RNA in human endometrium are increased by estrogen

Haining REB[1], Jones DSC[2], Schofield JP[2], Smith SK[1]
Department of Obstetrics and Gynaecology, University of Cambridge[1], MRC
Molecular Genetics Unit, Addenbrooke's Hospital, Hills Road, Cambridge, UK[2]

Estrogen causes proliferation of endometrium *in vivo* but it is not known if this is a direct effect or one mediated by other mitogens. Epidermal growth factor causes mitosis in many cell types and its receptor has been identified in all cell types of the human uterus. In the rat, estrogen stimulates expression of mRNA for the EGF receptor. In the mouse estradiol stimulates expression of messenger RNA for prepro EGF and the EGF precursor has been demonstrated by immunohistochemistry. The aim of this study was to investigate the expression of EGF in human endometrium and to determine the effect of estrogen on its expression.

The presence of EGF specific mRNA was demonstrated in human endometrium using the reverse transcriptase polymerase chain reaction. Total RNA extracted from endometrium was used to synthesize complementary DNA using oligo dT as the primer. To selectively amplify the cDNA encoding EGF a pair of oligonucleotide primers were designed which flanked the cDNA fragment encoding the mature EGF peptide. After 30 cycles of amplification the predicted 257 base pair PCR product was isolated by agarose gel electrophoresis. Partial sequencing by direct methods demonstrated that the sequenced PCR product was identical to the mature EGF coding region of human mRNA for the EGF precursor.

Total RNA was extracted from whole endometrium which had been stimulated *in vitro* with 10 nM estradiol in serum free medium for three hours alone. The RNA was analyzed using a dot blot technique in which the probe was a ^{32}p-end labelled oligonucleotide complementary to the EGF precursor RNA. Densitometry of the resulting autoradiogram revealed a 4-fold increase in steady state levels of EGF specific mRNA in estradiol-stimulated endometrium.

These findings demonstrate that EGF specific mRNA is expressed by human endometrium and that its expression is increased by estradiol.

Cell-specific metallothionein gene expression in mouse decidua and placenta

De SK, McMaster MT, Dey SK, Andrews GK
Department of Biochemistry and Molecular Biology, and Departments of Obstetrics
and Gynecology, and Physiology, Ralph L. Smith Research Center, University of
Kansas Medical Center, Kansas City, KS

Oligodeoxyribonucleotide excess solution hybridization, Northern blot and *in situ*
hybridization were used to analyze metallothionein gene expression in mouse decidua and
placentae during gestation. Metallothionein (MT) -I and -II mRNA levels were constitutively
elevated, 11- and 13-fold respectively relative to the adult liver, in the deciduum (D8), and
decreased coordinately about 6-fold during the period of development when the deciduum
is replaced by the developing placenta (D10-16). Coincident with this decline, levels of MT
mRNA increased dramatically in the visceral yolk sac endoderm. *In situ* hybridization
established that MT-1 mRNA was present at low levels in the uterine luminal epithelium
(D4), but was elevated at the site of embryo implantation exclusively in the primary decidual
zone by D5, and then in the secondary decidual zone (D6-8). Although low levels of MT
mRNA were detected in total placental RNA, *in situ* hybridization revealed constitutively high
levels in the outer placental spongiotrophoblasts. Analysis of pulse-labeled proteins from
decidua and placentae established that these tissues are active in the synthesis of MT. The
constitutively high levels of MT mRNA in decidua were only slightly elevated following
injection of cadmium (Cd) and/or zinc (Zn), whereas in placentae they increased several-
fold. MT mRNA levels were equally high in decidua and experimentally induced deciduomata
(D8) which establishes that decidual MT gene expression is not dependent on the presence
of the embryo or some embryo-derived factor. Although the functional role of MT during
development is speculative, these results establish the concept that from the time of
implantation to late in gestation, the mouse embryo is surrounded by cells, interposed
between the maternal and embryonic environments, which actively express the MT genes.
This suggests that MT plays an important role in the establishment and maintenance of
normal pregnancy.

Preimplantation embryo development in the mouse: role of epidermal growth factor

Paria BC, McPherson C, Dey M, Dey SK
Departments of Obstetrics and Gynecology and Physiology, University of Kansas
Medical Center, Kansas City, KS

The mammalian embryo during its preimplantation development undergoes a series of morphological and functional changes from a unicellular zygote to a differentiated blastocyst. Little is known about the control of growth and differentiation of the embryo during this period. Two distinct features during the preimplantation embryo development are activation and mitosis following fertilization of the egg and differentiation of the embryonic cells into inner cell mass and trophectoderm at the blastocyst stage. Preimplantation embryo development is unique in the sense that development up to the blastocyst stage can occur outside the reproductive tract, i.e. *in vitro* in simple balanced salt solution. Although the embryonic growth rate is slower *in vitro* and the number of cells of the *in vitro* grown blastocysts is smaller, these blastocysts appear to be physiologically normal as evidenced from delivery of healthy young following their transfer into a foster mother. The question is then how the mitosis and differentiation are controlled in the preimplantation embryo. It appears to be a function of autoregulation. A recent report indicates that the mouse preimplantation embryo expresses several growth factor genes and accumulates these growth factors (Science 241:1823, 1988). Thus, it could be hypothesized that the growth factors originating from the embryo or the reproductive tract might regulate the mitosis and differentiation of the preimplantation embryo in an autocrine/paracrine fashion.

If it is true that the preimplantation embryos produce growth factors which act on them, then it is conceivable that the preimplantation embryos cultured individually in a defined volume of culture media will show inferior development because of the greater dilution of the growth factors in the media secreted from individually cultured embryos as compared to those cultured in groups. However, this inferior development could possibly be corrected by the addition of exogenous growth factors. To test this hypothesis, 2-cell embryos (day 2 of pregnancy, day 1 = vaginal plug) were cultured individually or in groups (5 and 10) in microdrops (25 μl) under silicon oil in Whitten's medium under 5% CO_2 + 5% air in a humidified chamber at 37° C for 72 h in the presence or absence of epidermal growth factor (EGF). The embryos were examined every 24 h to monitor their development and growth. At the termination of the culture, blastocyst cell numbers were determined. Embryos cultured individually showed inferior development to the blastocyst stage (0/43 blastocysts at 48 h and 21/43 blastocysts at 72 h) as compared to embryo cultured in groups (groups of 5 embryos: 9/45 and 37/45 blastocysts at 48 h and 72 h, n = 9; groups of 10 embryos: 4/30 and 23/30 blastocysts at 48 h and 72 h, n=3). The inferior development of embryos cultured individually was dramatically improved by the addition of EGF in the media. Thus, while 2 ng/ml EGF did not improve considerably the number of embryos forming blastocysts (2/12 blastocysts at 48 h and 5/12 blastocysts at 72 h), higher doses of EGF (4, 10 or 200 ng/ml) showed a large increase in the number of blastocysts formed (4 ng: 4/16 and 13/16 blastocysts;

10 ng: 9/21 and 18/21 blastocysts; 200 ng: 10/27 and 24/27 blastocysts at 48 h and 72 h, respectively).

The results indicate that not only did the number of embryos developing to blastocysts improve, when cultured in groups, or individually in the presence of EGF, but also the time required for blastocyst formation was reduced. Furthermore, embryos cultured individually had fewer cell numbers (29.1 ± 4.0, n = 43) at the blastocyst stage as compared to those individually cultured in the presence of EGF (2 ng: 39.0 ± 6.9, n = 12; 4 ng: 71.0 ± 5.0, n = 16; 10 ng: 64.0 ± 6.0, n = 21; 200 ng: 52.1 ± 4.1, n = 27), or cultured in groups (group of 5 embryos: 55.6 ± 4.9, n = 9; group of 10 embryos: 72.6 ± 6.1, n = 3). The results suggest that growth factors are important for preimplantation embryo development and growth. although we do not know whether other growth factors are involved, EGF appears to play a vital role in preimplantation embryo development and blastocyst formation. EGF and transforming growth factor-α (TGF-α) mediate their functions through the same receptors. If TGF-α shows similar effects, then we can postulate that while TGF-α produced by the preimplantation embryo (science 241:1823, 1988) will promote embryonic development in an autocrine fashion, EGF of the reproductive tract origin (J Cell Biochem, in press) may do so in a paracrine fashion. This information could be of importance *in vitro* fertilization programs in the human. Further investigation is required to gain more insights into the role of growth factors in embryonic development.

Comparative study of antiviral and 2',5'-oligoadenylate synthetase inducing activities of trophoblast proteins of the pig and the cow

Short EC, Geisert RD, Fulton RW, Zavy MT, Helmer SD
Oklahoma State University, Stillwater, OK, USDA, ARS, El Reno, OK

Maintenance of corpus luteum (CL) function during early pregnancy in cattle and sheep depends on conceptus secretion of trophoblast protein-1 (TP-1). In contrast, CL maintenance in the pig appears to depend on conceptus secretion of estrogen. However, the porcine conceptus secretes a complex of polypeptides (pCSP) of similar M_r and pI to TP-1. Ovine and bovine TP-1 have extensive sequence homology to bovine α-interferon (α-IFN). How the close homolog of conceptus polypeptide with α-IFNs relates to its role in control and maintenance of pregnancy is unclear at present. IFNs also have the capacity to induce the cellular enzyme 2',5'-oligoadenylate (2-5A) synthetase. The 2-5A system, which includes 2-5A synthetase, 2-5A and a 2-5A dependent endoribonuclease is affected by virus infection, hormones and growth status of the cell as well as IFN. In addition to its antiviral role, the 2-5A system may be involved in control of cell growth and cellular responses to hormones. We therefore assessed the antiviral activity (AA) of bTP-1 and pCSP as well as their effect on 2-5A synthetase in MDBK and endometrial cells. We compared AA of bTP-1 and pCSP in uterine flushings and media from 24 h embryo culture. We also compared the ability of bTP-1 and pCSP to stimulate 2-5A synthetase activity in MDBK cells and in endometrium collected from cyclic and pregnant animals.

Uteri from cyclic (n = 35) and pregnant (n = 45) cows were flushed with saline on D 5-17 post-estrus. Uteri from cyclic (n = 27) and pregnant (n = 12) gilts were flushed with saline on D 9-18 post-estrus. AA in uterine flushings was assessed by inhibition of cytopathic effects of vesicular stomatitis virus in MDBK cells. AA is undetectable (<10 U) in flushings of cyclic cows and gilts. In pregnant cows, AA is first detectable on D 15 when conceptus length is 4 mm (4258 ± 61 U) increasing monotonically with time and conceptus size through D 17 when conceptus length is greater than 100 mm (AA 6.8×10^6 U). In pregnant gilts, AA is first detectable on D 14 (conceptuses length greater than 200 mm, AA 2110 ± 39 U), increasing to 5692 ± 46 U on D 16, and declining slightly (3713 ± 35 U) on D 18. Media from 24 h conceptus cultures, D 17 bovine (1 embryo each) and D 16 porcine (5-8 embryos each) contained 3.6 ± 1.4 and 0.14×10^6 U AA, respectively. Serial dilutions ($0.01-1 \times 10^3$ U AA) of bTP-1 and pCSP were examined for their capacity to induce 2-5A synthetase activity. Based on AA, capacity of bTP-1 to induce 2-5A is comparable to that of IFN-α and -β and is ten-fold higher than that of pCSP. *In vivo* endometrial 2-5A synthetase activity was measured in samples collected from cyclic (n = 25) and pregnant (n = 15) cows and from cyclic (n = 17) and pregnant (n = 12) gilts between D 0 and 18 post estrus. Endometrial 2-5A synthetase was similar between cyclic and pregnant cows from day 0 to 15. However, a four-fold increase ($p < 0.05$) in activity occurred in the gravid horn of pregnant animals on D 18 while activity of cyclic cows was unchanged. 2-5A synthetase activity of endometrium from cyclic and pregnant gilts did not differ throughout the period.

Although porcine conceptuses produce trophoblast protein it appears to be less active than bTP-1 in terms of both AA and capacity to induce 2-5A synthetase. Trophoblast proteins may participate in immunological protection of the embryo in both species, however, bTP-1 appears to function by way of the endometrial 2-5A system in maternal recognition of pregnancy in the cow. These results are consistent with the different signals for maternal recognition in the two species.

Hormonal regulation of metalloproteinase activity and extracellular matrix remodeling in human endometrial stromal cells in culture

Irwin JC, Gwatkin RBL

Reproductive and Developmental Biology, Research Institute, The Cleveland Clinic Foundation, Cleveland, OH

There is limited knowledge of the biochemical and cellular events that lead to the breakdown and shedding of human endometrial tissue during the normal menstrual cycle. To improve our understanding of the mechanisms of endometrial menstrual breakdown we studied the effects of progesterone withdrawal in serum-free cultures of human endometrial stromal cells. Treatment of steroid-free stromal monolayers with 30 nM estradiol (E2) + 300 nM progesterone (P) for 10 to 15 days induced multilayering and the production of a fibrillar extracellular matrix as seen by scanning electron microscopy. Analysis of the culture medium by electrophoresis in gelatin-impregnated acrylamide gels revealed one band of gelatinolytic activity (66 kD) in hormone treated cultures. After 2 to 5 days of hormonal withdrawal stromal multilayers underwent breakdown with dissolution of the extracellular fibers and shedding of superficial cells. Another band (62 kD) was detectable and the 66 kD species enriched in the culture medium of these hormone-withdrawn cultures. These biochemical changes were prevented by continued treatment of stromal cultures with P or other progestins, but not by treatment with P + the progestin antagonist RU486, E2, glucocorticoids, or androgens. Neither band was detectable in withdrawn cultures treated with the inhibitor of protein synthesis, cycloheximide (2 μg/ml). Proteolytic activity of both species was inhibited by the metalloproteinase inhibitor 1,10-phenanthroline (5 mM) but not by other protease inhibitors. The breakdown of stromal multilayers was prevented by the same hormones and biochemical inhibitors that showed an effect on proteolytic activity. Our results show that P-withdrawal induces changes in metalloproteinase activity that are correlated with the remodeling of extracellular matrix in human endometrial stromal cell cultures. These findings may be relevant to the mechanisms of tissue remodeling during the menstrual breakdown of the endometrium *in vivo*.

Contributors

G.K. Andrews, Department of Biochemistry and Molecular Biology, University of Kansas Medical School, Kansas City, Kansas

F.W. Bazer, Departments of Animal Science and Pediatrics, University of Florida, Gainesville, Florida

H.A. Bern, Department of Integrative Biology and Cancer Research Laboratory, University of California, Berkeley, California

D.D. Carson, Department of Biochemistry and Molecular Biology, The University of Texas M.D. Anderson Cancer Center, Houston, Texas

C. Chiappetta, Department of Pharmacology, University of Texas Medical School at Houston

D.A. Clark, McMaster University, Ontario, Canada

I. Damjanov, Department of Pathology and Cell Biology, Thomas Jefferson University, Philadelphia, Pennsylvania

S.K. De, Department of Biochemistry and Molecular Biology, University of Kansas Medical School, Kansas City, Kansas

S.K. Dey, Department of Obstetrics and Gynecology and Physiology, University of Kansas School of Medicine, Kansas City, Kansas

M. Edery, Department of Integrative Biology and Cancer Research Laboratory, University of California, Berkeley, California

R.M. Gardner, Department of Pharmacology, University of Texas Medical School at Houston

T. Iguchi, Department of Integrative Biology and Cancer Research Laboratory, University of California, Berkeley, California

A.L. Jacobs, Department of Biochemistry and Molecular Biology, The University of Texas M.D. Anderson Cancer Center, Houston, Texas

J.L. Kirkland, Division of Endocrinology, Department of Pediatrics, Baylor College of Medicine, Houston, Texas

L.A. Lavia, Department of Biological Sciences, The Wichita State University, Wichita, Kansas

T.H. Lin, Division of Endocrinology, Department of Pediatrics, Baylor College of Medicine, Houston, Texas

R.B. Lingham, Department of Pharmacology, University of Texas Medical School at Houston

D.S. Loose-Mitchell, Department of Pharmacology, University of Texas Medical School at Houston

M.T. McMaster, Department of Biochemistry and Molecular Biology, University of Kansas Medical School, Kansas City, Kansas

V.R. Mukku, Department of Pharmacology, University of Texas Medical School at Houston

L. Ogren, Department of Biology, Sinsheimer Laboratories, University of California, Santa Cruz, California

C.A. Orengo, Department of Pharmacology, University of Texas Medical School at Houston

N. Raboudi, Department of Biochemistry and Molecular Biology, The University of Texas M.D. Anderson Cancer Center, Houston, Texas

J.N. Southard, Department of Biology, Sinsheimer Laboratories, University of California, Santa Cruz, California

G.M. Stancel, Department of Pharmacology, University of Texas Medical School at Houston

F. Talamantes, Department of Biology, Sinsheimer Laboratories, University of Californea, Santa Cruz, California

G. Thordarson, Department of Biology, Sinsheimer Laboratories, University of California, Santa Cruz, California

P.-S. Tsai, Department of Integrative Biology and Cancer Research Laboratory, University of California, Berkeley, California

F.-D.A. Uchima, Department of Integrative Biology and Cancer Research Laboratory, University of California, Berkeley, California

U.M. Wewer, The University Institute of Pathological Anatomy, Copenhagen, Denmark

Index